DIETS
THAT WORK

Other books by Deralee Scanlon, R.D.:

The Wellness Book of I.B.S.

Other books by Larry Strauss:

What Do You Mean You Don't Want to Go to College?
(with Liliane Quon McCain)
When You Have Chest Pains (with Gershon Lesser, M.D.)
Financial Tips for Teachers (with Alan Weiss)

DIETS
THAT WORK

For Weight Control or Medical Needs

DERALEE SCANLON, R.D.
with **LARRY STRAUSS**

Lowell House
Los Angeles
CONTEMPORARY BOOKS
Chicago

ADVISORY

Not all diets are suitable for everyone and great care must be used in selecting a diet that is appropriate for you. The diets presented herein are in no way intended as a substitute for medical treatment or counseling. You should always consult a medical doctor before beginning any diet program.

The publisher and distributor of this book do not endorse statements, claims, or programs reviewed in this book. The publisher and distributor disclaim any liability, injury, or loss in connection with the diets set forth or the instructions and advice that appear in this book.

Library of Congress Cataloging-in-Publication Data

Scanlon, Deralee.
  Diets that work: for weight control or medical needs/by Deralee Scanlon with Larry Strauss.
     p. cm.
  Includes bibliographical references and index.
  ISBN 0-929923-40-5 : $19.95
  1. Reducing diets. 2. Diet therapy. I. Strauss, Larry. II. Title.
RM222.2.S2538 1991   91-12557
613.2'5—dc20   CIP

Requests for such permissions should be addressed to:

     Lowell House
     1875 Century Park East, Suite 220
     Los Angeles, CA 90067

Publisher: JACK ARTENSTEIN

Vice-President/Editor-in-Chief: JANICE GALLAGHER

Director of Marketing: ELIZABETH WOOD

Design: MIKE YAZZOLINO

Manufactured in the United States of America
10   9   8   7   6   5   4   3   2   1

To Demba and Ralph Scanlon, my parents, who taught me a life philosophy that included the principles of good nutrition so that I might set an example for others.

CONTENTS

FOREWORD   xv

HOW TO USE THIS BOOK   1

SECTION ONE: WEIGHT-CONTROL DIETS   7

TWELVE BASIC PRINCIPLES OF DIETING FOR WEIGHT MANAGEMENT   9

ORGANIZED PROGRAMS   15

    Overeaters Anonymous   16

    Take Off Pounds Sensibly (TOPS)   20

ENROLLMENT PROGRAMS   23

    Diet Center   24

    Jenny Craig   29

    Nutri/system   34

    Shapedown   40

    Weight Watchers   45

MEDICALLY SUPERVISED DIET PROGRAMS   53

    Health Management Resources   56

    MediBase   60

    Medifast   64

    Optifast   69

    Optitrim   74

    United Weight Control Corporation   77

    Weigh to Live   81

WEIGHT-LOSS BOOKS   85

    The Choose to Lose Diet   88

    The Executive Success Diet   94

The Feel Full Diet   99
The I-Don't-Eat (But I Can't Lose)
Weight-Loss Program   104
The I-Quit-Smoking Diet   108
Living Lean by Choosing More   115
The New American Diet   121
Not Another Diet Book   127
The Setpoint Diet   131
The Stop-Light Diet for Children   136
The T-Factor Diet   141
Winning Weight Loss for Teens   148
FOR THOSE WHO NEED TO GAIN WEIGHT   151
SECTION TWO: MEDICAL/HEALTH/SPECIALTY DIETS   153
ARTHRITIS   157
The Arthritis Relief Diet   159
CALCIUM ABSORPTION   165
Osteoporosis: Brittle Bones and the Calcium Crisis   166
The Calcium Connection   170
CHEMOTHERAPY   175
Nutrition for the Chemotherapy Patient   176
CHOLESTEROL REDUCTION   181
Controlling Cholesterol   183
Count Out Cholesterol   190
The 8-Week Cholesterol Cure   195
DIABETES   201
The UCSD Healthy Diet for Diabetes   203
FOOD ALLERGIES   209
The Allergy Discovery Diet   211
HYPERTENSION   217
Recipes for the Heart   218
HYPOGLYCEMIA   223
The Do's and Don'ts of Low Blood Sugar   224

INFLAMMATORY BOWEL DISEASE (I.B.D.)   229
    Eating Right for a Bad Gut   230
IRRITABLE BOWEL SYNDROME (I.B.S.)   235
    The Wellness Book of I.B.S   236
LACTOSE INTOLERANCE   243
    The Milk Sugar Dilemma   244
MULTIPLE SCLEROSIS (MS)   249
    The Multiple Sclerosis Diet Book   251
POST CORONARY   257
    An Affair of the Heart   258
WHEAT INTOLERANCE   263
    The Gluten Free Gourmet   264
CONSULTING A REGISTERED DIETITIAN   269
APPENDIX A: FOOD SOURCES OF IMPORTANT
           NUTRIENTS   271
APPENDIX B: RECOMMENDED DIETARY ALLOWANCES   273
APPENDIX C: METROPOLITAN LIFE INSURANCE COMPANY'S
           HEIGHT AND WEIGHT TABLES   275
APPENDIX D: REFERENCES TO SECOND OPINIONS   279

ACKNOWLEDGMENTS

WHEN I STARTED THIS BOOK, it was clear that in order to get through the necessary thousands of hours of research, I would need the cooperation of many people, some of whom would be strangers to me until I called on them for information. If, during the months of that process, I threw my hands up in frustration and weariness more than once, it is equally true that this project has introduced me to new friends and confirmed the strength of other, long-term friendships.

It has also given me a renewed appreciation for two groups of professionals in particular: *registered dietitians*, who are indeed the nutrition experts for both the public and others in the medical field; and *librarians*, whose remarkable efficiency and desire to serve must be appreciated by all authors. In both groups, there are too many to list individually here, but I will see to it that they know who they are.

Those people whom I must specifically thank in this space are: *Jack Artenstein*, my publisher, who conceived the idea for this book; *Larry Strauss*, for his skill at making often complex information clear and accessible to those who need it; my editor, *Janice Gallagher*, for judiciously knowing when to let me run with material and when to rein me in; *Lynn Wilcutts-Unroe, R.D.*, and *Jeann Young*, my dear friends, who provided valuable comments and suggestions; *Nils A. Shapiro*, whose help and encouragement in everything I do is a source of daily nourishment . . . and, finally, *Sterling* and *Star*, for their loving companionship.

Deralee Scanlon, R.D.

AUTHOR'S NOTE

HOWEVER YOU USE THIS BOOK *be sure to consult your physician* before beginning any diet. No one should treat any medical problem without the supervision of a qualified physician—and even then, you must be an active participant in your health. Everyone is unique, and a diet that may work for most people can have adverse side effects for some. No one can predict what will happen when an individual makes a radical change in eating habits, but by being an active and educated dieter, by working *with* your doctor, not passively putting yourself in his or her care, you can greatly reduce any potential risks. This is true whether the medical problem is obesity or a peptic ulcer.

A change in diet, whatever the reason for it, is never easy. Often, it means avoiding foods you are fond of. As a client once told me, it's like giving up an old friend. But it can also be a liberating experience, discovering that you *can* control what you eat and knowing the potential benefits.

Think of this book as an investment guide. The investment is in your life and your health.

FOREWORD

FOR YEARS WE'VE SEEN THE proliferation of new diets and diet plans guaranteed to shed pounds of fat better than any other preceding programs. The best seller list always has one or two celebrity diet books. New weight management treatment centers having "the latest and best programs" spring up in shopping malls around the country trying to deal with the pandemic of American obesity. And yet, throughout all of this, no clear concise assessment of the safety and effectiveness of these various programs has emerged. That is, until Deralee Scanlon's book, *Diets That Work.*

Ms. Scanlon is a registered dietitian with years of clinical experience in dealing with the challenges of the standard American diet. She brings this considerable experience to bear on evaluating the various diets and weight-loss programs that are currently available in the marketplace so that the consumer can make an informed choice about what really does work and what is mere marketing sizzle and hype.

I am most impressed with Ms. Scanlon's book, both for its accurate technical information and for its sensible and understandable summary of reasonable diet and weight loss expectations. By reading this book, you will learn not only about the safety and effectiveness of various diets that are now popular, but also about the whole contemporary concept of diet, weight management, and good health.

All of us who are working in this field recognize that weight management is a most complicated area in which to achieve long-term success. This is because of the complex nature of problems relating to eating and foods, which spill over into psychology, economics, self-esteem, personal history, metabolism, and lifestyle. Selecting a diet based on the evaluation process presented in *Diets That Work* can result in profound and positive changes in our relationship to food. This can lead to better food selection habits, which translates into successful weight loss and maintenance and better longterm health without having to depend on fads, crash programs, or products that only promote weight loss and regain.

I believe that this book makes a significant contribution to our understanding not only of which diets work but also of how and *why* they work.

Jeffrey S. Bland, Ph.D.

HOW TO USE
THIS BOOK

IN RECENT YEARS THE SCIENCE of nutrition has generated much information about how the foods we eat can affect not only our weight and the way we look but also our risk of major illness.

For weight loss alone, there are more than 17,000 different diet plans, products, and programs being promoted to Americans. Every year, we spend over $35 billion in our efforts to lose weight, and an ever-increasing amount of money in the pursuit of better health and increased longevity.

As a registered dietitian, I often work with people who are deeply concerned about their weight and about their health. Often, they are quite knowledgeable on the subject of diet and nutrition, well aware of the close connection between eating properly and the reduced risk of heart disease and other major illnesses, but they are also confused. There is plenty of accessible health information—on television and radio, in newspapers, magazines, books, and pamphlets—but there is also some outright *mis*information from product advertisers.

Your health and personal appearance, your physical comfort and self-image are too important to leave to chance. You need to know that the diet you choose is effective, realistic, safe, and right for you. It is no secret that most so-called fad diets offer little or no hope of long-term success, but some diets *do* work. Whether your objective is weight loss, weight gain, or the management of a specific medical problem, you can successfully attain your goal, provided you have the desire and the knowledge to help you do so.

The experiences of my private practice and the questions I have answered by mail, in my newspaper column, and on television and radio have led me to the firm conviction that people not only *want* concise, correct, and usable information; they have a real *need* to know. They should also understand that the word *diet* has a broader meaning than simply a regimen for weight management. *Diet* refers to everything a person eats and drinks at any time, whether or not it follows a plan and is meant to achieve a specific goal. Furthermore, those diets that do have a specific purpose are not limited to weight loss. Many medical conditions require changes in daily diet, although part of the treatment for these conditions often necessitates weight loss.

With that in mind, this book examines a number of diets that have, in my opinion, proved most effective. This does not mean there are no other diets or programs that work, but it does mean that you can feel confident about selecting one of the diets described here.

The information in these pages is the result of extensive research, including interviews with spokespersons—dietitians as well as company executives—from various diet programs along with a detailed and methodical analysis to ensure that each diet faces an equal challenge of whether it is, in fact, a diet that *works*. The primary criteria used to make this assessment were *effectiveness*—does the diet enable the dieter to accomplish his or her goal and maintain it?—and *adherence to the principles of good nutrition.*

Use this book as a permanent resource guide to help enrich your understanding of diet and nutrition, and to help you select which diet is right for you—the one that best suits your personal tastes, objectives, and budget. You will understand how and why it works so that you can achieve optimum results.

The range of diets includes not only those for effective weight control, but also those widely prescribed for specific health conditions, among them: diabetes and hypoglycemia; heart disease, hypertension, and cholesterol control; irritable bowel syndrome (IBS) and colitis; arthritis; wheat and lactose intolerance; and food allergies.

Each diet or program profile is formatted for easy access, so that you can readily find out what you need to know when you need to know it. This format will address (where applicable) the following questions about each diet:

NAME OF PROGRAM OR BOOK In addition to the name, information about joining the program or buying the book (national headquarters address and telephone number, or publisher and date of publication) will be included.

BACKGROUND   An informed dieter is a dieter with an edge. The more you know about a diet before taking the plunge, the better prepared you are to benefit from it. Knowledge of how the diet came to be or about the background of its founder or author can lend important insight. In cases of books, this heading will be titled, *About the author(s)*.

WHOM IT'S FOR   Many diets are designed for individuals with specific problems or objectives. A diet can work only if it is the right kind of diet for the particular dieter.

HOW IT WORKS   Ignorance is not bliss when it comes to dieting. The more you know about how a diet works, the better you are able to make that diet work for you.

NUTRITIONAL EVALUATION   Diets that work utilize sound principles of nutrition and biochemistry, some to a greater degree than others. Dieters need to know exactly how sound the science behind a prospective diet is, and also what the overall health effects of the diet are. The nutritional assessment of each diet will look at both macronutrients (those nutrients that comprise the greatest amount of dietary intake: carbohydrates, protein, and fat) and micronutrients (vitamins and minerals). These assessments are based upon a variety of well-known scientific criteria, such as those of the National Academy of Science, the American Heart Association, and the American Cancer Society.

Discussion of nutrient content will often refer to the recommended dietary allowances (RDAs) of the Food and Nutrition Board of the National Academy of Sciences National Research Council. Listed below is the recommended macronutrient caloric breakdown of a diet—that is, what percentage of daily calories should come from carbohydrates, what percentage from protein, and what percentage from fat. It is important to note that U.S. dietary goals were updated in 1989 from this:

Carbohydrates.....................................50% to 60%
Protein..15% to 20%
Fat ....under 30%

to this:

Carbohydrates.....................................55% to 65%
Protein..10% to 15%
Fat ....under 30%

Some of the diets in this book do not reflect this recent change, but I do not consider this a significant problem. As long as fat remains under 30 percent or less, a 5 percent swing in protein and carbohydrate does not undermine the effectiveness of a diet. Weight loss diets are meant as temporary modifications and thus need more flexible standards. Moreover, weight loss diets with total calories as low as, for example, 1,000 a day, should probably *not* reflect the recommended lower percentage of protein, since that could lead to a protein deficiency.

(It should be pointed out here that some obesity authorities—including the highly-respected Dr. George L. Blackburn of New England Deaconess Hospital—disagree with the generally accepted protein guidelines and claim that a higher daily protein level of approximately 70 grams is required in order to preserve lean muscle tissue . . . especially on medically-supervised, very-low-calorie programs.)

I will also refer to how well these diets provide essential micronutrients (vitamins and minerals). Following are the current Recommended Dietary Allowances (RDAs) (also modified in 1989) for daily intake by healthy adults. (For more specific guidelines based upon age, sex, height, and weight, see Appendix B.)

VITAMINS

VITAMIN A

| Males | 800 retinol equivalents (RE) |
| Females | 800 RE |

VITAMIN B-1 (THIAMINE)

| Males | 1.5 milligrams (mg) |
| Females | 1.1 mg |

VITAMIN B-2 (RIBOFLAVIN)

| Males | 1.7 mg |
| Females | 1.3 mg |

VITAMIN B-6 (PYRIDOXINE)

| Males | 2.0 mg |
| Females | 1.6 mg |

VITAMIN D

| Males | 200 International Units (IU) |
| Females | 200 IU |

VITAMIN E

| Males | 10 mg |
| Females | 8 mg |

VITAMIN K

| Males | 80 micrograms |
| Females | 65 μg |

FOLATE (FOLACIN)

| Males | 200 μg |
| Females | 180 μg |

VITAMIN B-12

Males	2.0 μg
Females	2.0 μg

NIACIN

Males	19 mg
Females	15 mg

VITAMIN C

Males	60 mg
Females	60 mg

Pantothenic acid, another essential vitamin, has no official RDA; 4 to 7 mg, however, is generally considered a safe and adequate range.

MINERALS

CALCIUM

Males	800 mg
Females	800 mg

PHOSPHORUS

Males	800 mg
Females	800 mg

IODINE

Males	150 μg
Females	150 μg

SELENIUM

Males	70 μg
Females	55 μg

IRON

Males	10 mg
Females	15 mg

ZINC

Males	15 mg
Females	12 mg

MAGNESIUM

Males	350 mg
Females	280 mg

Potassium, another essential mineral, has no official RDA; 1,600 to 2,000 mg, however, is generally considered a safe and adequate range.

In addition to the above vitamins and minerals, there are accepted daily recommendations for cholesterol (300 milligrams or less), sodium (2,400 milligrams or less), and fiber (20 to 30 grams).

You will notice that in many diets some nutrients are less than 100 percent of the RDA but above two-thirds of those amounts. Two-thirds of the RDA, while not ideal, is nevertheless safe and adequate and will not, according to the National Academy of Sciences, lead to nutritional deficiencies. In any event, the RDAs are intended to serve as "yardsticks" for adequate nutrient intake, rather than as strict minimums.

COST   Weight control and overall good health are invaluable commodities, but it never hurts to know how much cash a program is likely to take.

PRACTICALITY   Beyond the financial cost, diets can place many other demands on the dieter. Issues of convenience are important for some people. Certain issues of practicality can mean the difference between a diet that is realistic for a particular individual and one that is simply unworkable.

LIFESTYLE AND EXERCISE   Diets and diet programs are about more than calories and food groups. Diet is only a part of any successful approach to weight control or disease management. Most diets that work recognize that nutritional recommendations are meaningless unless accompanied by methods of changing lifestyle to accommodate changes in diet. Many successful diets also recognize the vital role of exercise.

WHY IT WORKS   If you're wondering "Why *these* diets?" here is where you will find out. The effectiveness of any diet has to do with a number of factors, and it is important to understand them. It is like knowing the end of a movie before it starts: it makes the story easier to follow.

POTENTIAL DRAWBACKS   Even diets that work may not be perfect. Knowing the flaws in advance can help you avoid them and ensure success.

SECOND OPINION   Matters of judgment deserve more than one voice. While most of these second opinions are not contradictory, they do shed additional insight.

Because of the book's format, it may not be necessary for everyone to read the entire book at once. Many of you can refer to specific sections as needed. However, most of the diet plans, while intended to address preexisting conditions (obesity and diabetes, for example), also suggest *preventive* dietary measures. Thus, if you are concerned about the potential of future illness because of your family medical history or other known risk factors, you may want to examine the corresponding section as part of a *preventive* health regimen.

SECTION ONE

WEIGHT-CONTROL DIETS

WEIGHT-CONTROL DIETS

TWELVE BASIC PRINCIPLES OF DIETING FOR WEIGHT MANAGEMENT

ACCORDING TO A SURVEY conducted by the Caloric Council, one of every four American adults is dieting at any given time. Of those people, 97 percent cut down on high-calorie foods, 88 percent exercise, 29 percent skip meals, 12 percent crash diet, and 4 percent use diet pills. How many of these dieters reach and maintain their weight loss goals? Unfortunately, not many—otherwise, the number of Americans on diets would steadily dwindle to nothing!

In his official report on nutrition and disease, C. Everett Koop, then–U.S. Surgeon General, told America what medical researchers and dietitians have known for years: "Improper diet is associated with five of the ten leading causes of death in this country, including heart disease, cancer, strokes, diabetes and atherosclerosis, a hardening of the arteries. . . . Approximately 34 million adults—one-quarter of the population—are significantly overweight. . . . It is recommended that Americans achieve and maintain a desirable body weight through sensible diet, increased exercise and reduced intake of salt and alcohol."

The decision is yours and the means are available. The goal of this section is to help you find the weight management program best suited to your needs. But before we delve into the diet and program profiles, here are 12 general and universal elements of any successful weight management system. Many of these ingredients also apply to medical diets.

1. YOU MUST TRULY WANT TO SUCCEED. Whether your motivation is to live a healthier, longer life or simply to look and feel better, reaching and maintaining an ideal weight depends upon a strong desire. It must be a priority.

2. YOU MUST EAT HEALTHFULLY.   Your body needs a variety of nutrients from a balanced diet that includes all the food groups. Malnourishment (depriving your body of needed nutrients) is not the solution to excess weight or any other health problem. Malnourishment *is* a health problem—and even a person who is overweight can be malnourished.

Reducing caloric intake must, therefore, go hand-in-hand with proper nutritional food choices. When selecting a diet, pay attention to its nutritional breakdown. In order for a weight management program to be effective, *it must provide your body with all essential nutrients*. This is why I have rated the nutritional viability of the diets in this book.

Your commitment to losing weight must coincide with a new commitment to eating healthfully; the nutritional breakdowns of diets that help you lose weight may very well be much better than what you are currently eating.

3. LOSE WEIGHT AT A REALISTIC AND SAFE PACE.   Except in medically advised situations (and that does *not* include an impending swimsuit season), crash diets of fewer than 1,000 calories per day are the least effective way to lose weight and keep it off. Since a crash diet does not establish anything resembling a regular and satisfying regimen or promote good eating habits, it makes future maintenance of weight loss very difficult (about *three times* as difficult, according to a recent study by the chief of the nutrition/metabolism lab at the New England Deaconess Hospital in Boston). The body does not react well to sudden and extreme deprivation. In the absence of regular aerobic activity, crash dieting causes the burning of lean muscle tissue and the eventual replacement of that muscle tissue with fat. It also slows down your metabolic rate, so that your body burns calories more slowly and then regains fat more quickly.

Losing weight gradually allows you to eat in a way that will help you reach *and then maintain* your ideal weight and achieve an acceptable percentage of body fat—15 to 25 percent for men; 20 to 28 percent for women. Gradual weight loss allows your body to adjust to the change and, through physical activity, rebuild lean muscle tissue.

The ideal rate of weight loss is generally considered to be 4 percent of body weight per month or an average of 1 to 2 pounds per week for most people. This means that for every 100 pounds you weigh at any given time, it is recommended you lose no more than four pounds in the following month. This recommendation is in keeping with a new study, entitled *Toward Safe Weight Loss*, conducted by the Michigan Health Council. (For exact calculations, multiply your weight times .04).

CURRENT WEIGHT	RECOMMENDED MONTHLY WEIGHT LOSS
150 lbs.	6 lbs.
175	7
200	8
225	9
250	10
275	11
300	12

Losing weight at this rate can reduce the potential health risks, but nothing can entirely eliminate them. As with any other radical body change, weight loss achieved in any manner has its perils. In most cases, however, the dangers of weight loss are far less threatening than the long-term hazards of remaining overweight except that certain degrees of rapid weight loss require medical supervision.

4. YOU MUST CHANGE ANY BAD EATING HABITS.   Following an appropriate diet is a start, but it isn't enough. You must *adopt* that diet—make it a habit, not an exception.

If people were to eat only when their bodies were truly hungry and in need of fuel, few if any of us would have a weight problem. People eat for many reasons, only one of which is real bodily hunger. People use food to pacify themselves when bored, stressed-out, depressed, or lonely. Social situations can also put food in your mouth when your body doesn't need any. How many times have you been at a party or restaurant and eaten simply because the food was there, or because eating was expected of you?

Changing eating habits is a great challenge, but never underestimate your ability to grow and change. Make change your priority and it will happen.

5. MAKE COMPLEX CARBOHYDRATES THE STAPLE.   Fruits, vegetables, legumes (peas, beans, lentils), and whole grains are the best sources of energy and a key to successful weight loss. Your body runs on the glucose that is best derived from these foods. You need protein too, but in smaller amounts, and your dietary fat needs are even smaller.

While all excess calories turn to fat, the rate at which they do so differs drastically. For example, to convert 100 excess calories of carbohydrates into fat storage, your body uses about 23 of those calories, leaving only about three-quarters to be turned into body fat. To convert 100 calories of dietary fat into fat storage, in contrast, your body only uses 3 calories—leaving 97 percent to be converted.

With the exception of very-low-calorie *medically supervised* diets, the diets that work generally use complex carbohydrates as the primary food.

6. DRINK LOTS OF WATER.   Studies show that an increase of water intake can reduce body-fat deposits. Water is needed to enable the kidneys to function properly in filtering waste. When the kidneys are not working to full capacity, the liver is forced to help out by doing part of the job. The liver then becomes less efficient in one of its jobs: burning stored fat into usable energy—and the result can be slower weight loss.

Diets that work are even more effective when you drink a minimum of eight glasses of water per day.

7. YOU MUST HAVE SOME KIND OF PHYSICAL ACTIVITY IN YOUR LIFE.   A change in diet by itself may not enable you to achieve or maintain an ideal weight. The body's metabolism (the rate at which it burns calories for fuel) is designed for optimum survival. That means *the less food you eat, the slower your body will utilize that food.*

This design may have been great for our prehistoric ancestors for whom food was often scarce and body fat was a necessity for austere times. They ate wild animals that were lower in fat than the domestic livestock eaten today, and by necessity they led very active lives. Today, for many people, food is readily available, highly processed, high in fat, and many of us lead lives with little physical activity. Today, in a world in which excessive body-fat storage often means discomfort, frustration, social condemnation, and health problems, the body's survival mechanism can work against our objectives: cutting down on calories may *not* result in the long-term loss of excess weight.

It is possible to circumvent this system—to get the body to metabolize quickly while cutting down on caloric intake. One is exercise.

Daily exercise not only raises the body's metabolic rate; it uses fat as its fuel source (if it is aerobic), raises the level of HDL (high-density lipid) good cholesterol (especially in men), helps to control appetite, builds lean muscle tissue, improves muscle tone, and releases into the body chemical endorphins that can enhance your general sense of well-being.

Exercise need not involve miles of jogging or complex aerobic routines or competitive sports, but it must cause you to exert energy for a sustained period of time. For some, a brisk one-mile walk is all that is needed. Consult your physician to learn your own personal appropriate level of exercise.

8. TAKE A VACATION FROM DIETING.   Many dieters encounter the problem of weight plateaus; they lose weight to a point and then, without departing from their diet, get stuck at a level. These plateaus are often caused by the body's desire to "defend" its set point (the weight your metabolism is geared to maintain). This usually happens more quickly with chronic dieters. According to Dr. John Foreyt, director of the Nutrition Research Clinic at Baylor College, "the gradual cessation of weight loss is the real danger for dieters." Dr. Foreyt further points out that plateauing produces "feelings of hopelessness and despair, which lead to more abusive dietary habits. One's self-esteem is just destroyed in the process."

A study by Dr. George L. Blackburn of Harvard Medical School suggests that the body is somehow designed to lose weight for no longer than twelve consecutive weeks—and anyone trying for longer is apt to encounter frustration and the danger of failure—but that after a brief "rest" period of several months, the body will readjust and be able to lose weight for up to another twelve-week period.

9. SET A REALISTIC WEIGHT LOSS GOAL.   Without a realistic goal, dieting can be a frustrating and demoralizing endeavor. It is always helpful to see the light at the end of the tunnel, but if your goal is not realistic, that light will be elusive.

Unless your physician has instructed you to reach a specific weight objective, it is up to you to set a target. Setting a realistic weight loss goal does not have to mean deciding to the exact pound how much you wish to weigh. Some people succeed when they set small goals, enabling them to gain confidence as they approach their ideal weight. Others want to be able to know, at any given time, how far along they are on the journey to maintenance.

Most people can simply picture the weight at which they will look and feel their best—the weight at which their clothes feel most comfortable and at which they are likely to receive the greatest number of compliments. This can be an effective approach, but a word of caution: in envisioning the weight at which you will look and feel your best, do not consult the pages of *Vogue* or *GQ* or any other magazine. *Your best* is yours and yours alone! Utilize your imagination to create a conception of what *you* will look like and, perhaps more importantly, to consider how you will *feel*, inside and out.

10. EAT SLOWLY.   It takes approximately 20 minutes for your brain to "turn off the hunger button" and let your body know that you have eaten enough to satisfy your appetite. If you eat too quickly, you are likely to finish an entire meal before you have had a chance to realize you didn't need that much.

11. DON'T SKIP MEALS.   If too much time elapses between meals—say, more than three or four hours—your blood sugar level will drop and you may very well overeat at the next meal, more than making up the difference in calories. It's best to spread meals throughout the day, ideally three small meals and two snacks—all totaling no more calories than you would usually eat in three "regular" meals.

12. CHOOSE A DIET THAT WORKS FOR YOU.   That is what the rest of Section One of this book is about: finding the plan that best enables you to adhere to the first eleven basic principles of dieting for weight management. Each of us has unique needs and unique problems, which is why this book reviews an assortment of diets and other weight management programs that vary biochemically, philosophically, and economically. As you read on, try to imagine yourself following the various diets and weight management programs until you can clearly envision yourself at your ideal weight emerging from one of them.

WEIGHT-CONTROL DIETS

ORGANIZED PROGRAMS

THESE ARE ORGANIZATIONS founded for the sole purpose of helping people with eating disorders and/or weight problems to overcome their destructive behavior and to lose the necessary weight through strength of fellowship with people who have similar problems.

These are not diet programs per se. They view overeating and being overweight as problems more complex than simply choosing what foods to eat. Through strength in numbers—in group support and compassion—members strive to achieve control over their eating, their weight, and their lives in general. Members may use any effective eating plan (such as those recommended later in this book) in tandem with group affiliation.

OVEREATERS ANONYMOUS

World Service Office
P.O. Box 92870
Los Angeles, California 90009

(213) 542-8363

BACKGROUND This program began 30 years ago when three women started meeting in order to apply the principles of Alcoholics Anonymous to their dieting problems. There are 10,800 chapters in 60 countries and approximately 150,000 members nationwide in this nonprofit organization.

WHOM IT'S FOR Overeaters Anonymous (OA) is a self-help group for compulsive overeaters: people who use food the way an alcoholic uses liquor. OA publishes a questionnaire to help people determine whether that description fits them.

The goal of the OA program is to help its members abstain from eating compulsively. Weight loss is therefore an accompanying benefit of the program. OA views compulsive overeating as an illness that can be controlled—in their words, "arrested"—but not cured. The only requirement for membership is a desire to stop compulsive overeating. OA members include compulsive overeaters who are overweight as well as those who are not.

It should be noted here that not every overweight person is a compulsive overeater. Some people are overweight because of lack of exercise, improper diet (*what* they eat, not *how much*), or various illnesses and other conditions that can affect the metabolic rate. For anyone who *is* a compulsive overeater, however, OA can be a life-saver. In addition to the regular program, OA offers slightly modified meetings for young people.

HOW IT WORKS The OA Tools of Recovery form a 12-step program almost identical to that of AA, with food and compulsive overeating replacing alcohol and drinking. The 12-step philosophy suggests that compulsive overeating is a symptom of emotional and spiritual deficit, which must be confronted once the compulsive eating itself has ceased. The steps include admitting powerlessness over food and turning your life over to a higher power of your own choosing (anything from a generalized God to a personal God to the strength of the group itself). Helping other OA members is one of the cornerstones of the program, and OA's long-term successful members are virtually unanimous in saying that service to others is crucial to their own abstinence from compulsive overeating.

Abstinence from compulsive overeating is defined by the individual for himself or herself, although the generally accepted rule of thumb is: no more than three moderate meals per day. OA members follow any of a number of available diet plans or their own doctor-recommended weight loss program in conjunction with OA membership. It is possible to combine OA membership with one of the diet programs recommended in these pages. Some OA members, especially those new to the program, find it useful to write down, or phone in to another OA member, their food plan for each day. Like Alcoholics Anonymous, OA adheres to the principle of taking recovery one day at a time.

OA meetings are held periodically; in most large cities you can find at least one every night of the week. Meetings are led, usually in a rotating fashion, by recovering members who have achieved at least 21 days of abstinence from overeating. Meeting formats vary, including:

—*Discussion meetings* involve members in problem solving, program clarification, and conferences on relevant topics, including the twelve steps and twelve traditions of the program.

—*Pitch meetings* provide opportunities for members to briefly share their experiences as compulsive overeaters—what they were like, what OA has done for them, and what they are like now.

—*Speaker meetings* feature recovering members sharing their "experience, strength, and hope" in more extended format.

—*Beginner meetings* are smaller, more intimate question-and-answer sessions to help newcomers.

—Step study meetings devote themselves to a study of each of the programs steps and traditions; participants share their experiences as related to each step.

—Literature meetings feature the reading and discussion of a chapter from *Overeaters Anonymous*, the book on which the program is based.

Although there is no mandatory attendance, members are encouraged to attend in order to share "experience, strength, and hope" with other recovering compulsive overeaters.

Each member is encouraged to have a sponsor, an abstaining OA member in whom to confide on a one-to-one basis. Newcomers are told, "Find someone who has what you want [presumably in terms of successful control of eating] and let him or her help you get there, too."

There is no such thing as failure in OA. Members know firsthand what it is like to grapple with abstinence from compulsive overeating; they encourage those who slip back into destructive eating habits to hope for the future rather than live in regret about the past.

Some OA members resolve to completely abstain from what they consider to be their particular problem foods, those they believe they *cannot* eat in moderation. Some members, for example, believe that refined sugar is to them what alcohol is to the alcoholic. This is not a belief of OA as a whole. OA, in fact, takes no positions on good foods or bad foods. There are no lectures on dieting, nutrition, or exercise—although, some members will tell you, "Most of us are experts already, since we've tried and failed at every diet there is!" No weigh-ins or food diaries are required.

The heart of the program is anonymity, which creates an atmosphere of equality and respect, and which allows freedom of expression without censorship, criticism, or gossip.

NUTRITIONAL EVALUATION   Because OA recommends no specific food plan, there are no nutritional data to evaluate.

COST   Donations are requested, but there is no formal fee or dues structure. There is no additional food expense inherent in the program.

LIFESTYLE AND EXERCISE   Since OA believes that compulsive overeating is the symptom of an illness, there is no structured behavior modification, though group support and inspiration provide opportunities for radical changes in eating habits. Most members concur as to the relative ease of traveling or dining in a restaurant while adhering to the program.

Exercise is not a part of the program, and thus should be pursued through other means.

WHY IT WORKS   The group support helps members overcome the feeling that they are alone with their overeating problem, and member success stories provide added motivation to keep on trying. The 12 steps of AA have worked for millions of otherwise doomed alcoholics. Why shouldn't they work for compulsive overeaters? The buddy system provides not only encouragement, but a social network for those in need as well.

Successful OA members boast not only that their eating and weight are under control but that their lives are happier and more productive. OA's anonymity and freedom are attractive for many overeaters, encouraging personal responsibility and integrity.

POTENTIAL DRAWBACKS   The OA group leaders and those asked to be sponsors are not trained and therefore are not equipped to deal with anyone who has serious psychological problems. Since the OA program is based on mutual support and equality, it offers a freedom that can be troublesome for those people who need a rigid structure to follow.

Take Off Pounds Sensibly (TOPS)

TOPS International Headquarters
4575 South Fifth Street
P.O. Box 07360
Milwaukee, Wisconsin 53207-0360

(414) 482-4620

BACKGROUND   TOPS is a nonprofit organization founded in 1948 by Esther S. Manz, a housewife who overcame her weight problem through the mutual support of friends with a common goal. With the success of Manz and her friends, their weekly meetings grew in popularity; the rest is history. There are now more than 12,000 chapters of TOPS in the United States and Canada—at least one in every state and over 700 in California, with more than 18,000 members in that state—and in 20 other countries worldwide.

WHOM IT'S FOR   TOPS defines itself not as a program for compulsive overeaters but for anyone who wants to lose weight sensibly for any reason. They believe that there is strength in numbers and in the camaraderie of individuals coming together with a common mission, and that this strength is just what it takes for many people to reach and maintain their ideal weight.

HOW IT WORKS   This is not a diet program; it is a lifestyle approach to weight management. The focus is on the inspiration derived from group meetings, which are referred to as "continuing education." They are held at a regularly scheduled time each week and usually last an hour and a half.

Each meeting begins with members weighing in to have their progress recorded. Then roll call is taken and each member stands and announces his or her weight loss or gain. After each member has testified, the entire chapter's total pounds lost (minus those gained) is announced. The remainder of each meeting is devoted to a program referred to as "therapy." These programs address issues of sensible and safe weight loss and weight management, including the emotional pitfalls of losing weight.

Some meetings feature nonmember professionals as speakers. Dietitians are often asked to speak to TOPS meetings about a variety of health-related weight-management topics. In keeping with the organization's nonendorsement policy, speakers are forbidden to promote products of any kind.

At other meetings, group discussions are led by an elected leader. Discussions are conducted with the following stipulation: Speak *to* your fellow members, not *at* them. Because each chapter of TOPS is self-directed by elected members, programs vary. Members are encouraged to maintain group strength and connectedness by communicating over the phone between meetings.

To enhance group morale, TOPS publishes a monthly membership magazine, *TOPS News*, which includes success stories, low-calorie recipes, and a Q&A column. TOPS also holds contests and recognition programs that acknowledge and reward those who have successfully lost weight and maintained that loss. There are numerous yearly TOPS retreats and one yearly convention where members can enjoy a quiet vacation and receive continual support as well as practical advice.

TOPS provides no standard food plan and encourages members to have their personal physicians prescribe realistic weight goals, eating plans, and schedules for losing weight. In the absence of medically prescribed dietary advice, TOPS urges a prudent and sensible diet of approximately 1,200 calories per day.

NUTRITIONAL EVALUATION   Because TOPS recommends no specific food plan, there are no nutritional data to evaluate.

COST   Annual membership fees are $12 in the United States and $17 in Canada. Each chapter also has its own dues, averaging about 50 cents a week. The first meeting you attend is free.

LIFESTYLE AND EXERCISE   While not professionally administered, the TOPS program promotes behavior modification through the exchanges at weekly group support meetings. Although not a part of the TOPS program, exercise of a safe—and, where necessary, medically supervised—nature is highly recommended, and TOPS members generally seem aware of the importance of physical activity in connection with a change in diet to achieve and maintain weight loss.

WHY IT WORKS   The program's motto is "I care"—and for any-one struggling with overweight, those two words can be profound. Group support has been shown to be a highly effective behavioral modification tool for many people, and the emphasis on success gives struggling members hope for the future. They can look at the long-term maintaining members, called KOPS—Keeping Off Pounds Sensibly—and say, "If they can do it, so can I!"

Low membership fees make the program accessible to almost everyone and probably help to maintain group harmony. In the spirit of optimism, TOPS donates some of its membership dues to fund the Obesity and Metabolic Research Program, which investi-gates causes and potential remedies of obesity.

POTENTIAL DRAWBACKS   There is a lack of program unifor-mity among the various chapters; new members may find it neces-sary to visit a number of chapters in order to determine if this program is for them. Since group leaders are elected from among the members (rather than hired professionals such as psychologists or dietitians), members must rely on faith for the good intentions and common sense of their fellows.

WEIGHT-CONTROL DIETS

ENROLLMENT PROGRAMS

THESE ARE PRIVATE BUSINESSES designed to make money in exchange for helping people lose and maintain weight. The monetary aspect does not in itself lessen the potential effectiveness of a program—in fact, some people take these programs more seriously precisely because of the financial investment involved. But you have to bear in mind the profit motive. While most enrollment programs offer support and counseling, they are limited by the realities of business: the counselors are paid employees and the meter is ticking. They may be genuinely concerned about your plight, or they might just be doing their job, reciting from a memorized script without much feeling or interest.

On the other hand, enrollment programs are comprehensive. They not only offer a support system, they also provide nutritional counseling, a diet, and, in some cases, most or all of the actual food.

Keep in mind that, as with all businesses, these programs are subject to changes in format and cost.

DIET CENTER

921 Penn Avenue
9th Floor
Pittsburgh, Pennsylvania 15222

(800) 333-2581

BACKGROUND   For years, Sybil Ferguson had repeatedly lost and gained weight, much of it from crash dieting, until she discovered (when she was scheduled for surgery) that she was malnourished. Consequently, she researched healthy eating concepts, consulting with her physician until she had worked out her own healthy weight loss program, on which she lost more than 50 pounds. Wanting to share her success with others, she founded Diet Center in 1970; two years later the first franchise was established. There are now 2,300 Diet Center franchises in the United States, Canada, Australia, England, Singapore, Bermuda, and Guam.

WHOM IT'S FOR   Diet Center is for virtually anyone who can afford the moderate financial investment and who wants intensive one-on-one counseling along with a fairly rigid food program. Diet Center requires the approval of a physician for anyone under 10 years old, anyone with a medical condition requiring medication, or anyone with more than 50 pounds to lose. The Center sends progress reports to the M.D. and requires further medical evaluations after each 40 pounds of weight loss, to ensure the health of the client.

For children and adolescents, Diet Center offers youth programs based upon age, height, and weight, with higher caloric levels to allow for physical growth.

HOW IT WORKS   Prospective clients have an initial meeting with a Diet Center counselor to discuss weight problems and goals using Metropolitan Life Insurance Company's table of ideal body weight ranges (see Appendix C).

Those who join are encouraged to commit themselves to an intense involvement with the Center and its diet counselor, including daily weigh-ins. They are asked to visit the center every day of the week except Sunday (although Diet Center has become more flexible in order to accommodate people for whom daily visits are impossible). The program does not require that clients purchase Diet Center foods (except for supplements); dieters buy their own food from structured menus.

The program consists of four phases, each with its own meal plans.

Phase One: Conditioning lasts two days and is intended to detoxify and cleanse the body and to stabilize the blood sugar. Food intake during this phase is high in protein (10–12 ounces per day); high in fruits (five to seven servings daily), vegetables (unlimited), and grains (two servings per day); low in simple carbohydrates or sugars; and low in fat (two teaspoons of oil per day). Along with the meal plans, Diet Center clients must take four tablets a day of the Diet Center food supplement tablets (35 calories of soy protein, fructose, dextrose (sugar), B-vitamin complex with four grams of protein, and five grams of carbohydrate), which, according to the company, stabilizes the blood sugar.

At some Diet Centers,* new clients are given a body composition analysis to determine their ratio of lean muscle mass to fat and basal metabolic rate. The client's program will be based on this data. These tests are also given after the second week and every fourth week thereafter, and necessary dietary modifications are made accordingly.

During this phase and throughout the program, Diet Center encourages dieters to drink eight 8-ounce glasses of water daily, a key factor in good digestion and maximum weight loss.

Phase Two: Reducing continues for 12 weeks or until the client's weight loss goal is reached. The diet is lower than the first-phase diet in protein (seven to nine ounces), lower in fruits (two servings per day) and vegetables (two large servings: three cups raw, one to two cups cooked); and about the same in grains (two servings) and oil (two teaspoons). Dairy, plus a wider variety of such foods as potatoes, barley, pasta, and rice, were added to this phase in 1990.

In addition to the allowable food, dieters continue to take four Diet Center supplement tablets per day. The meal plans add up to a

---

*More than half the centers are now equipped for this procedure and, according to a Diet Center spokesperson, they intend to make this feature standard.

minimum of 945 calories per day for women and a minimum of
1,300 calories per day for men, including 35 from the supplement
tablets. As in all phases, Reducing involves daily counseling and a
daily weigh-in, though exceptions are made for clients with special
circumstances.

Phase Three: Sta-b-lite is a nine-week program of increased calories—1,240 to 1,465 per day for women, 1,240 to 1,725 for men. This
phase is divided into two parts. For the first three weeks, the daily
diet is 12–14 ounces of a protein source, two to four large servings of
vegetables, one fruit serving, two grain or cereal servings, and one
cup of dairy products. For the next six weeks, protein is reduced to
seven ounces for women and nine ounces for men. During this
entire phase clients are given one Sta-lite bar daily (a blood-sugar
stabilizer high in fiber and natural sugar, fortified with vitamins and
minerals). One-on-one counseling is reduced to three times per
week.

Phase Four: Maintenance lasts for one year and provides six
different calorie levels from 1,395 to 2,585 that are based upon body
composition, activity level, height, and dieters new weight. This
gives the individual a wider variety and larger quantities of food
each day, with unlimited raw vegetables plus two to four cups of
cooked vegetables, seven to nine ounces of protein, three to five
fruit servings, two to eight cereal and grain servings, two table-
spoons of oil, and two cups of dairy products. Visits to the Center
are reduced to once a week. Image One classes, which run throughout the entire program concurrent with the various phases, now
focus on utilizing the tools learned earlier in the program.

NUTRITIONAL EVALUATION   The weight loss phase of the program has the following nutritional distribution:

	Women	Men
Carbohydrates	50%	44%
Protein	27%	31%
Fat	23%	25%
Sodium	850 milligrams	
Fiber	25 to 30 grams	

The carbohydrate levels for men are lower than national pre-
1989 dietary goals, and the protein is high for both men and women,
though fat remains within these same national goals.

COST   The cost depends on the amount of weight to be lost. Here is a general idea:

Lifetime membership: $50 to $75

Reducing phase: $35 to $50 per week

Sta-b-lite phase: $35 to $50 per week

Maintenance: $100 (refundable if you stay within five pounds of goal weight for one year)

To lose approximately 30 pounds over a 12-week reducing period, the overall cost would total from about $885 to $1,225.

PRACTICALITY   Diet Center offers a line of five frozen main-dish foods along with 70 other food products, including spices, seasonings, crackers, beverage mixes, and salad dressings. These products are not mandatory. All of the required foods can be bought at any supermarket. The Conditioning and Reducing Phase supplements, however, are available only at Diet Centers, and only to clients during those two phases. Some Diet Center locations also offer recipe preparation classes, tasting sessions, and a Diet Center cookbook.

The recommended daily visits to a Diet Center may be difficult for many working adults to schedule, but the large number of locations means that the trip is often a short one.

Since dieters choose their own foods from among the meal plans, clients claim that the program is relatively easy to follow while traveling or eating out.

LIFESTYLE AND EXERCISE   Weekly behavior modification classes, called Image One, cover nutrition and stress management. The program counselors, who follow a uniform format created at company headquarters, are successful Diet Center graduates. They attend periodic training classes at headquarters but are not required to have any professional training in nutrition or psychology.

Diet Center encourages exercise but does not provide formal exercise classes. They do offer exercise tapes.

WHY IT WORKS   Diet Center, which reports an average weekly weight loss of three pounds for women and four pounds for men, offers dieters an opportunity to immediately begin to replace bad eating choices with good ones. Unlike most enrollment programs, Diet Center allows dieters to shop for all of their food and prepare it themselves. This kind of supervised independence can be invaluable; it can be the beginning of a lifetime of weight control through good food choices. The menu plans are nutritionally sound and flexible enough to suit a wide variety of tastes.

Diet Center also offers a great deal of personal support from counselors and weekly group classes so that when the going gets rough, there is often someone there to help.

POTENTIAL DRAWBACKS   The daily weigh-ins can create negative reinforcement and frustration. Successful weight loss normally includes occasional small daily weight fluctuations—usually from fluid retention—which should not be dwelt upon.

The somewhat restrictive diet (in types and amounts of allowed foods) may undercut the important concept of balanced eating. Nutrients are most effective when derived, as much as possible, directly from the foods in a balanced diet that includes all food groups—with supplements acting as a kind of nutritional insurance.

There are some peculiarities of this program from a nutritional point of view. For example, since protein is higher, carbohydrate levels are lower for men than in the nationally recommended goals; and legumes (such as peas, beans, and lentils) are banned from the Reducing phase, although they are low in fat, high in fiber, and a good source of protein. This was a decision made by the founder.

Finally, as is true of most weight loss organizations, counselors are not required to be registered dietitians.

When I questioned the need for the Diet Center's food supplement tablets, a spokesperson for the company explained that, since fluctuating blood sugar levels can produce hunger and weakness, the supplement is considered an "insurance" against low blood sugar. The fact is that if dieters don't skip meals, and follow the menu plans, this additional supplementation (and its cost) would seem to be unnecessary.

JENNY CRAIG

445 Marine View Avenue
Del Mar, California 92014

(619) 259-7000

BACKGROUND   This weight loss chain was founded in 1983 in Australia by businesswoman Jenny Craig and her husband, Sid. They selected Australia to launch their program because at the time there were few weight loss centers in that country. There are now 100 Jenny Craig centers in Australia along with 10 in New Zealand, 30 in England, and more than 450 in the United States. Prior to this venture, the Craigs paid their dues in the weight loss business by operating (and learning from) a much less successful chain of centers in Southern California called Body Contours.

WHOM IT'S FOR   This program is for anyone with at least 10 pounds to lose who can afford the substantial cost and who is looking for a plan that is both well-structured and promotes independence. Jenny Craig does not accept people with multiple food allergies and lacks special provisions for those with lactose intolerance (the inability to digest milk sugar) or gluten intolerance (the inability to digest wheat protein). Jenny Craig does, however, have a special program for children and adolescents (ages 8 through 17).

HOW IT WORKS   The initial meeting includes a computerized calculation of the new member's projected weight loss schedule, based on the individual's caloric intake and the amount of weight to lose. Jenny Craig estimates the average weekly weight loss of its clients at one to two pounds for women and two to three pounds for men.

The Jenny Craig diet offers a variety of weekly meal plans at approximately 1,000 daily calories for women and 1,200 for men. Meal plans are interchangeable, provided that exchanges are of equivalent caloric levels. The program includes a multiple vitamin and mineral supplement to ensure adequate nutrition.

Most of the food is provided by Jenny Craig in the form of frozen, pre-plated microwaveable entrees; shelf-stable reheatable foods; canned items such as chili, soups, and pasta dishes; and snack foods including mousse, popcorn, and peanut butter snack bars. The Jenny Craig food must be supplemented with fresh fruits, vegetables, breads, crackers, and cereals, and dairy products such as milk, yogurt, and cheese.

During the first half of weight loss, clients eat only Jenny Craig foods every day. During the second half, clients decrease their reliance on the company's foods, using them only five days a week. The other two days consist of supermarket foods from menu plans with an assortment of food exchange categories; fruit, for example, is listed in varying quantities of uniform caloric content.

By the ninth week of the weight loss phase, dieters follow menu plans without any of the Jenny Craig foods. The shift from prepackaged food to meal planning is gradual, giving clients time to learn and adjust along the way—and hopefully to prepare for a lifetime of maintenance.

Once the dieter's goal weight is achieved, caloric levels are adjusted for weight maintenance, calculated as follows:

For women: goal weight times 13 (a standard activity factor). For example, a woman with a goal weight of 120 pounds would be given a maintenance level of 1,640 calories per day.

For men: goal weight times 15.

In either case, there is a minimum caloric level of 1,200.

The Jenny Craig diet program includes various group and one-on-one sessions designed to provide support and behavioral modification. During the weight loss phase, dieters attend weekly 20-minute sessions with their counselors (trained Jenny Craig employees, not registered dietitians). They are also required to attend a weekly 40-minute lifestyle class, where groups of 10 to 15 people share success stories, watch informational videotapes, and get answers to their questions.

NUTRITIONAL EVALUATION The women's 1,000 calories per day and men's 1,200 are distributed as follows:

Carbohydrates	60%
Protein	20%
Fat	20%
Sodium	2,000 milligrams
Fiber	15 to 18 grams

The Jenny Craig diet conforms to generally recognized health goals except for fiber, which is low. The 20% protein is acceptable when combined with both high carbohydrates and low fat levels as is the case here. The sodium level is in keeping with national goals. Jenny Craig's diet is also within health goals for cholesterol—100 milligrams per 1,000 calories. The company's multiple vitamin and mineral supplement assures 100 percent of the RDAs for all important nutrients.

COST   Current Jenny Craig prices include:

One-time registration fee: $79 (dropouts are permitted to return to the program without repaying this fee)

Jenny Craig foods (three meals and three snacks per day): $65 per week

Supplemental vitamins: $2.35 per week

Maintenance: $99 for one year

Additional home lifestyle counseling tapes: $75

The approximate cost of this program comes to $40 per pound, or about $1,200 to lose 30 pounds. This amount varies somewhat according to such factors as the dieter's adherence to the program.

PRACTICALITY   This program is fairly flexible, making it attractive to people with demanding lives, such as single working parents and traveling executives. Jenny Craig foods are readily available at the company's locations and may be purchased once a week when the client attends a counseling session. Classes are offered at various times of day, six days a week.

As for eating out, Jenny Craig recommends that during the first half of weight loss, when the company's entrees must be eaten every day, dieters should eat the Jenny Craig cuisine at home; then, at the restaurant, order a salad and noncaloric beverage. When a client reaches the halfway point in weight loss, Jenny Craig provides a *Dining Out Guide* to help in the appropriate selection of restaurant foods during the days when the dieter is not eating the Jenny Craig cuisine.

Traveling Jenny Craig clients may attend meetings and counseling sessions and pick up food at any Jenny Craig center in any state. As an alternative, the company can supply two-week menus of take-along foods that do not require refrigeration.

LIFESTYLE AND EXERCISE   The Jenny Craig program features one-on-one counseling with company-trained leaders who have at least a bachelor's degree in a related field, such as psychology or nutrition.

The weekly Lifestyle group sessions include videotapes developed by Dr. Morton Shaevitz, a behavioral psychologist at Scripps. These videos present information on nutrition, psychology, and exercise. Discussions follow each video presentation so that clients learn how to apply the information to everyday situations. They also receive behavioral homework assignments to enhance independent development.

Weight loss maintenance includes monthly weigh-ins and lifestyle classes. According to Jenny Craig, these classes are based on the work of Alan Marlet, a Ph.D. in relapse prevention at the University of Washington. The maintenance program uses the concept of Moderation Mountain, a triangular emblem with a person inside symbolizing the dieter balancing the three outside forces of his or her life: human control, no control, and total control (which refers to obsessive behavior). Each month's meeting has a different theme. December's meeting, for example, might focus on coping with holidays, while July's might be about summer barbecues and eating during vacations.

There are no formal exercise classes or facilities, but the company rigorously encourages dieters to do some sort of physical activity. Walking is generally recommended as the first step for the recently inactive. A walking program is offered on two 60-minute audio cassettes. Jenny Craig's exercise booklet, titled "F.I.T.T.," emphasizes the importance of aerobic exercise and provides information about target heart rate, warm-up and cool-down procedures, and resistance training guidelines.

Clients choose an exercise plan and keep a record of daily physical activity along with a daily food diary, which is reviewed by the nutrition counselor.

WHY IT WORKS   The Jenny Craig foods are conveniently packaged and easily prepared and the program encourages dieters to make their own food choices early in the dieting process. This enables clients to learn good eating habits and to be responsible for the control of their portion sizes. This puts an early emphasis on behavior modification as an integrated part of weight loss and weight management, which is reinforced during the one-on-one counseling sessions and lifestyle classes.

POTENTIAL DRAWBACKS Jenny Craig's nutrition counselors are not required to hold degrees as dietitians. As a result, their knowledge may be limited to the nutritional facts of the Jenny Craig program.

Finally, busy people may find the twice-a-week meetings inconvenient and also may neglect to supplement the Jenny Craig food with fresh fruits, vegetables, and grains—leaving their diet unbalanced and lacking in many vital nutrients.

JENNY CRAIG'S YOUTH PROGRAM Jenny Craig offers a 12-week program for children and adolescents from 8 to 17. Behavior modification is a strong component of this program, which addresses such issues as self-esteem and peer pressure. Weight goals are based on growth charts, and clients are encouraged to grow into their proper weight and to develop healthy eating habits. To that end, the young participants plan their own menus from guides in which foods are divided into three categories of caloric content; A-foods are low calorie; B-foods are medium; C-foods are high. The clients are given adult guidance to ensure that they select balanced eating plans.

Fast-food eating and other practical concerns are addressed, and the program suggests what it calls Champion Choices for such potentially troublesome situations as dinner at Wendy's—for example, a hamburger, baked potato, and milk rather than a cheeseburger, french fries, and a soda. Emphasis is placed on choices and responsibility. If the young dieter wants a high-fat meal, he or she must be responsible for limiting consumption of other high-fat foods for the rest of that day.

NUTRI/SYSTEM

3901 Commerce Avenue
Willow Wood Office Center
Willow Grove, Pennsylvania 19090

(800) 321-THIN

BACKGROUND In 1971, a Philadelphia businessman named Harold Katz consulted with nutritionists and a medical doctor in an attempt to help his mother lose weight. The resulting weight loss program soon became a family business called Shape-Up. A year later the name was changed to Nutri/system. Katz contracted with various manufacturers to produce foods under a private label—first canned, then frozen, freeze-dried, and ready-to-heat pouches. In 1986 the company was sold to its current owner and CEO, Don McCulloch. At the time of this writing, Nutri/system's national medical director is Stuart H. Shapiro, M.D., who is assisted by a registered dietitian.

Nutri/system is probably the best-known and most financially successful of the enrollment-style diet programs, with about 2,000 company-owned and franchised centers in the United States and Canada, Australia, England, and France.

WHOM IT'S FOR This program is for anyone who is over 14 years old, at least 10 percent above ideal body weight, who has at least seven pounds to lose and wishes to lose them in a medically safe way. Nutri/system does not accept pregnant women or anyone on antidepressant medication or diuretics. Enrollees must be able to afford the substantial cost and be comfortable with the program's lack of dietary independence. Nutri/system is especially attractive to those who don't want to keep a food diary, count calories, or weigh food portions.

No physical exam is required for enrollment, but an M.D.'s approval is required if there is a serious medical condition such as diabetes, heart disease, kidney disease, anorexia, or bulimia. Nutri/system's 340 menu variations can accommodate most food preferences, including those of vegetarians or persons with lactose or gluten intolerance.

HOW IT WORKS   The program begins with a tour of the Nutri/ system center, followed by a health history and lifestyle/weight loss profile questionnaires (the latter developed by a psychologist). From these answers a computer-generated food program is tailored to the individual's needs.

The Nutri/system diet is built around its own private-label pre-packaged meals, referred to as Crave-Free Meal Plans. There are 100 meals to choose from—either microwaveable, in reheatable pouches, or freeze-dried and prepared by adding water. The meal plans are adaptable to a number of diet-restrictive medical conditions. A diet of approximately 1,000 to 1,500 calories consists of three prepackaged meals and three snacks. The program allows for unlimited amounts of low-calorie vegetables, as well as two fruits and one cup of a starchy vegetable from company-provided food lists. Clients are advised to drink a minimum of eight glasses of water per day.

During the weight loss phase of the program, clients eat Nutri/ system foods every day, making their choices for the coming week from printed menus. Clients are weighed in once a week. According to Nutri/system, the results average a loss of one and a half to two pounds per week—a safe and manageable rate, adhering to national weight loss guidelines. There are also weekly 15-minute meetings with diet counselors. These "nutritional specialists" are not usually registered dietitians; they are Nutri/system employees trained to answer common nutritional questions about the program. Weekly 30-minute group meetings called Behavior Breakthrough sessions, teach such things as basic food exchanges and portion control, and continue until weight loss is achieved.

During the maintenance phase of the program, which begins as soon as the goal weight is achieved, clients eat Nutri/system foods twice a week. On the other five days they eat supermarket foods according to an individualized caloric program ranging between 1,500 and 2,500 calories per day. Each plan has prescribed numbers of servings per food group.

Nutri/system offers one year of supervised maintenance, which includes weekly meetings with a nutrition specialist and a behavioral counselor for the first two months. This is followed by twice-a-month meetings for months three through six, and once-a-month meetings for the last half of the year of supervised maintenance.

NUTRITIONAL EVALUATION　According to Nutri/system, the 1,000 to 1,500 calories per day offer a balance of all important nutrients. The caloric breakdown is as follows:

```
Carbohydrates ........................... 60%
Protein .................................. 24%
Fat ...................................... 16%
Sodium .................................. 2,400 milligrams
Fiber ................................... 24 grams
```

These percentages will promote weight loss. The protein level is a little high—15 to 20 percent was the pre-1989 recommended goal—but since the diet is only 1,000 calories, a higher protein percentage is usually necessary to ensure against a protein deficiency. In general, this diet should support good health by its combination of high complex carbohydrates and low fat. Aside from protein, this diet conforms to nationally accepted pre-1989 nutrition goals; Nutri/system claims that the Crave-Free Meal Plan itself meets the standards of the National Research Council's pre-1989 RDAs. I would add that anyone eating only 1,000 calories on *any* program should probably consider a vitamin and mineral supplement (not to exceed 100 percent of the RDAs) in order to ensure all of the essential nutrients. Nutri/system's program provides such a multiple vitamin and mineral supplement.

COST　Program costs vary, depending on the time necessary to achieve the desired weight loss. The fee structure is as follows:

Basic program cost: $250–$600 (rates differ among the various centers)

Crave-Free meals during weight loss phase: $70–$75 for the first week (which includes some optional foods in addition to the "regular food pack") and $59–$66 per week from the second week on, up to maintenance

Crave-Free meals during yearlong maintenance: about $12.50 per week

The total cost for a 30-pound weight loss is approximately $1,700–$2,000.

PRACTICALITY   Since the program includes the use of special Nutri/system food, proximity to the nearest center has a lot to do with how practical it is for you. Assuming that you live or work close to a Nutri/system center, the Crave-Free meals are user-friendly—they require no weighing or measuring and only the most basic preparations. Having to supplement them with fresh produce and nonfat milk from the market, however, means a minimum of two stops to shop for food. For anyone who is responsible for pre-paring meals for a spouse and/or children, the Crave-Free meals may actually be an inconvenience, since there will be multiple meals to prepare each night.

Travel may or may not be a problem. Nutri/system members may attend meetings or pick up Crave-Free meals at any of its 2,000 locations throughout the United States, Australia, England, France, and Canada. But this doesn't help if you're planning a safari in Kenya, or even a Caribbean cruise. Nor is it of much use if you're staying in a motel room without a kitchen.

Eating out is difficult. No restaurants, as yet, include Crave-Free meals on their menus, and few people want to endure the embarrassment of handing a microwaveable tray to a waiter and asking to have it heated up. In this respect, the cost of the pro-gram may be largely offset by the money saved by not eating in restaurants.

LIFESTYLE AND EXERCISE   The weekly Behavior Breakthrough sessions are designed to help clients with the behavioral aspects of losing weight. The group format of the meetings is helpful, since it can create a sense of camaraderie and peer support, although the bonds are not likely to be as strong as those in either TOPS or OA. The staff conducting these sessions are neither fellow dieters nor professional behavior therapists nor usually registered dietitians; their only requirement is a bachelor's degree in psychology. Some of these staff members may be very knowledgeable, personable, and even inspirational to clients, but there is no guarantee of that, and the value of the sessions is a somewhat unpredictable variable.

Nutri/system offers no formal exercise classes, but its Body Breakthrough activity program encourages exercise on three levels:

1. Everyday activities (such as standing while talking on the telephone)

2. Walking

3. Low-impact aerobics (a tape is provided)

Designed by Stanford University researcher Dr. Peter Wood, this program is intended to help overweight clients become more active, encouraging regular activity schedules.

WHY IT WORKS   Nutri/system allows the dieter the freedom to select from a fairly wide variety of meals. Foods are flavor-and texture-enhanced for increased satisfaction and to help prevent feelings of dietary deprivation. In addition to flavorful meals, Nutri/system sells packaged flavor enhancers in response to the Duke University Obesity Clinic's research finding that dieters have an exaggerated need for flavor and texture.

Nutri/system offers a financial incentive for success: if you complete the yearlong maintenance program without regaining more than five pounds, Nutri/system will reimburse you up to half of your basic enrollment fee (a refund of $150–$200). If you drop out before reaching your weight loss goal but rejoin within the time frame originally projected for that goal, you do not have to repay the enrollment fee.

POTENTIAL DRAWBACKS   When I made surprise visits to several Nutri/system centers, posing as an interested client, I was given no information about the program, not even a descriptive brochure, until after I had completed a multipage questionnaire and health history and set up an appointment to see a counselor. This practice is obviously a tool to help Nutri/system sell memberships, but it is a disservice to prospective clients, many of whom are in an uncomfortable and vulnerable position and might prefer to make a decision based on facts alone and not on a strong sales pitch.

Since Nutri/system mandates use of its own prepackaged food during the entire weight-loss phase, the program *does not* initially enhance the client's understanding of the responsibility for proper food choices.

Nutri/system's claim of having a health professional on site at each location can be somewhat unreliable. Several surprise visits to Nutri/system locations found some with registered nurses or other health professionals, and some without any.

Finally, a number of people on the Nutri/system program have encountered gallbladder disease—some so serious that their gall-bladders had to be removed (a class-action lawsuit is pending). I should point out, however, that scientific research has found that any weight loss diet presents a risk of gallbladder disease for people who have a great deal of weight to lose. Thus, the high number of such cases for Nutri/system may be as much a reflection of the organization's large enrollment as anything else.

Shapedown

Weight Management Program for
Children and Adolescents
Balboa Publishing Corporation
11 Library Place
San Anselmo, California 94960

(415) 453-8886

BACKGROUND This program was founded in 1979 by Laurel M. Mellin, M.A., R.D., director of the Center for Child and Adolescent Obesity at the University of California at San Francisco School of Medicine. It was developed by Mellin and other faculty members at the school's Department of Pediatrics and Family and Community Medicine. The program is currently used in over 450 hospitals and clinics and by several hundred private practitioners. Shapedown graduates number more than 60,000.

WHOM IT'S FOR Shapedown is for children (ages 6 to 12) and adolescents (13 to 20) who are obese, have an eating disorder, or are trying to improve their fitness and eating habits. Parents are required to concurrently join the Parent Program to ensure family involvement and support.

Adolescent obesity is no small problem. According to a recently published study, 75 percent of American teenagers have tried dieting, and at least 20 percent currently suffer from obesity. If you have an overweight adolescent child, I cannot overemphasize the importance of dealing with the problem *now*.

Increasing research evidence suggests that one's weight during adolescence has a significant impact on adult weight. An obese 12-year-old has a one-in-four chance of becoming a normal-weight adult; an obese adolescent has only a one-in-28 chance of becoming a normal-weight adult. Several studies confirm that some form of comprehensive intervention for adolescent obesity can produce significant long-term improvement, not only in weight, but also in food and exercise attitudes, blood pressure, total cholesterol level, serum triglyceride level, and, perhaps most important of all, self-esteem.

HOW IT WORKS   The adolescent program is 12 weeks long. It uses no set diet and does not exclude any foods, but rather aims to improve the teenager's dietary habits. Foods are divided into four categories:

- Free foods are those with less than 30 percent of their calories from fat, less than 10 percent of their calories from simple carbohydrates (sugars), and containing fewer than 30 calories per serving.

- Light foods are those with less than 30 percent of their calories from fat, 10 percent of their calories from sugars, but higher in overall calories than free foods.

- Heavy foods derive more than 30 percent of their calories from fat or more than 10 percent of their calories from sugars.

- Junk foods are mostly fat, high in calories, and offer little nutritional value.

Program participants are encouraged to eat foods primarily from the free and light categories, but not to the complete exclusion of the other two so that they do not feel too deprived.

According to Shapedown, most adolescents set a weight loss goal of one pound per week. Rigid or very-low-calorie diets are discouraged so that weight loss is gradual and does not decrease the teenager's growth, burn an excess of lean muscle tissue, or create nutritional deficiencies.

The overall goals of the program are a positive lifestyle change in the adolescent and improved self-esteem, in addition to long-term weight loss and maintenance—not only for the sake of appearance and general well-being but also to reduce the future risk of major diseases associated with obesity, such as diabetes, heart disease, and certain forms of cancer.

A major component of the Shapedown program is educational, working to increase the adolescent's knowledge of nutrition, exercise, physiology, and weight management principles. Each Shapedown client is given an easy-to-read teen workbook, entitled *Just for Teens!* and is personally supervised by a physician, dietitians, and licensed exercise and mental health professionals. Yet Shapedown encourages self-directed change; along with their parents, participants make self-assessments throughout the program, choosing and revising their own goals and strategies. Strategies may include monitoring, role playing, imagery, visualization, decision making, and cognitive restructuring.

Parents and adolescents attend separate counseling sessions. Parents are encouraged to change the entire family's diet to include lighter and more nutritious foods, and to increase family activity time and exercise. Parents are also counseled in numerous methods of effective parenting, including listening techniques for improved family communication, the use of verbal contracts or agreements for increased understanding and accountability, the setting of limits, the providing of enhanced emotional support, and the general promoting of family closeness.

At the same time, the *Shapedown Parent Guide* addresses the parents' feelings, provides coping strategies, and ultimately works toward a mutual parent/adolescent understanding that shifts the responsibility for weight to the adolescent, with the parent in a more supportive, rather than supervisorial, role.

Shapedown's children's program began seven years after the adolescent program. The philosophy, goals, and content are similar; the food summary and parent guidelines are the same. The children's program is 10 weeks long rather than 12 and features more direct parental involvement in the meetings and other on-site activities.

NUTRITIONAL EVALUATION   Since Shapedown dispenses no specific diet, there is no specific nutritional breakdown. Their nutritional advice is based on the U.S. dietary goals (see Appendix B).

COST   The average cost for the 10-week children's program or the 12-week adolescent program is $225. There are no special foods, supplements, or other extras.

PRACTICALITY   The program is easily adaptable since it allows the individual and family to set their own limits, goals, and strategies for weight loss and maintenance. The recommended foods are easily purchased at supermarkets and found in most restaurants, making dining out and traveling relatively easy.

LIFESTYLE AND EXERCISE A variety of techniques are applied to the behavioral problems of the child or adolescent. Clients are taught ways to distinguish real hunger from emotionally triggered cravings. They learn to identify emotional, sensory, social, and situational cues that trigger overeating patterns and then to find coping strategies.

Together with the professional staff, dieters work out ways to break the cycle of overeating and learn methods for dealing with negative and difficult emotions. They explore stress management, assertiveness skills, and relaxation techniques and are taught ways to develop a support system of friends and family members.

Exercise is a major component of the program. Clients learn to calculate their target heart rates and develop individual exercise programs, building on the components of fitness: endurance, flexibility, and strength. Dieters are encouraged to engage in any form of safe exercise that interests them—from walking to karate to modern jazz dance. Shapedown provides an "Exercise Summary" booklet with specific recommendations. The weekly meetings include exercises.

WHY IT WORKS Shapedown promotes family interaction and group support as the most important means of coping with the problems of childhood and adolescent obesity rather than focusing on strict meal patterns, food restrictions, or deprivation-style eating habits. Clients participate fully in designing their own regimen, rather than having something forced upon them. The exercise component of the program has been well researched.

All Shapedown staff who provide direct services to the public are thoroughly trained; they are required to complete an intensive course in adolescent obesity sponsored by the UCSF Center for Child and Adolescent Obesity. Because of this rigorous training and the scientific research behind the program, Shapedown has been praised in the *Journal of the American Dietetic Association* in a 1987 article entitled, "Adolescent Obesity Intervention: Validation of the Shapedown Program." Shapedown was given an award for excellence in consumer education from the National Food & Drug Association in 1988 and was recognized in 1989 by the American Medical Association as "an exemplary health promoting program."

POTENTIAL DRAWBACKS There is no ongoing national evaluation of Shapedown instructors to ensure uniformity of presentation skills and knowledge. After the initial 40 hours of training, providers of the plan are required only to be members of the Center for Child and Adolescent Obesity, from which they receive a quarterly publication. Thus, there is no certainty that these providers—although they are all health-care professionals—are delivering a universally standardized level of quality. In other words, some providers may be better than others.

WEIGHT WATCHERS

500 North Broadway
Jericho, New York 11753

(516) 939-0400

BACKGROUND The program was founded in 1961 by Jean Niedich, a homemaker seeking to manage her own weight control problems. Today, Weight Watchers is located in every major U.S. city (and many small ones) and in 23 foreign countries. In the United States alone, about 19,000 weekly meetings are held. Weight Watcher Centers are now partially franchised, although some remain company owned.

WHOM IT'S FOR Weight Watchers proclaims itself a lifestyle program, not just a diet plan. Thus, it is not for the quick-fix dieter, but for people who have accepted the concept that weight control is an ongoing problem that must be handled on a long-term basis. The program accepts anyone over 10 years old who is at least 10 pounds overweight.

HOW IT WORKS Weight Watchers uses a balanced, low-calorie food plan with a wide range of choices along with support-group meetings and helpful literature. The program goal is a gradual weight loss of between three and five pounds the first week and one to two pounds per week thereafter. As with all diets, men will tend to lose weight faster than women because they tend to have more lean muscle tissue and, therefore, burn calories faster.

Each member sets his or her own realistic weight goal based on Metropolitan Life Insurance weight charts, then determines at what rate he or she wants to lose it on the Personal Choice Program.

The Personal Choice Food Plan offers a three-level variety. These levels represent differing degrees of restrictions regarding the amount of food and flexibility. Members are encouraged to select from one of the three levels based upon their weight-loss goals and lifestyle needs, which involve stress level and social activity. Weight Watchers provides a questionnaire with a color-coded scoring chart to determine at which level the dieter should begin. Highly motivated members who want to achieve the fastest weight loss are usually assigned Level 1; Level 2, a moderate weight loss plan, offers an increase in flexibility in food choices (most members utilize this one); for slow and steady weight loss, Level 3 gives the widest variety and largest amount of food possible (while still promoting weight loss).

	LEVEL 1	LEVEL 2	LEVEL 3
Women	1,040 calories	1,200 calories	1,450 calories
Men	1,440	1,600	1,910
Youths	1,530	1,690	2,090

Dieters are required to stay on the selected level for at least one week. After that, they can retake the questionnaire and switch levels (the dieter can make this change every week, if necessary). This flexibility enables the dieter to tailor a program that best suits his or her lifestyle and makes weight loss as easy as possible.

Within each level, the diet organizes foods into six food group lists—dairy, fat, protein, vegetables, bread, and fruit—from which daily menus are derived. At each meal, the dieter is allowed a specified number of portions from each of these lists. These portions are logged into a food diary so that dieters can calculate their daily and weekly food intake totals. Those foods high in saturated fat and cholesterol are limited.

An additional miscellaneous category provides optional foods not on the other six lists, including sugar, honey, syrup, chocolate, cookies, and frozen yogurt. These are grouped in specific portion sizes by their caloric level. These lists also account for fast foods and other combination foods (those which contain more than one food item from differing lists such as cheese tortellini with tomato sauce).

Weight Watchers provides food diaries to assist in recording food choices; diaries from the first three weeks also contain sample menus. This organization also makes available a modified diet for members who need to overcome weight loss plateaus or who want to maintain a partial weight loss while taking a break from dieting.

Weight Watchers urges all dieters to eat three meals and consume six to eight 8-ounce glasses of water per day. The program also emphasizes the group strength and insights derived from its meetings. The most common types follow:

Traditional community groups are weekly 45-minute meetings held at 7 P.M. Members pay an $11 meeting fee and are weighed in, the data recorded confidentially. They receive program materials and recipes at each meeting and then engage in a group discussion. For the sake of standardization, discussion topics are identical at every Weight Watchers meeting throughout the world. These discussions are led by Weight Watchers members who have lost at least 10 pounds, maintained the loss for at least six weeks, and have attended an eight-week training workshop. The discussions are informal, with members sharing success stories and insights into what works for them.

Commuter meetings, weekly half-hour sessions held at 5 P.M., are a slightly abbreviated version of the traditional community groups.

At-work programs are weekly meetings scheduled during employee lunch breaks at various participating companies. Length of the meetings varies. Some companies pay for part or all of the program cost for their employees in advance; others reimburse employees once they have completed an 8-to-10 week program or have achieved their goal weight.

Community programs are designed for small towns of fewer than 5,000 people which might not otherwise be able to support a Weight Watchers chapter. The community program consists of 10 weeks of meetings, paid for in advance rather than on the usual pay-as-you-go basis. A minimum of 20 people is required. The meeting formats are similar to those of other Weight Watchers groups.

When dieters reach goal weight, they receive a maintenance plan booklet. The booklet contains information about eating and weight control, suggestions for dealing with common maintenance challenges, problem solving techniques, and a food dictionary (an expanded list of foods allowed on maintenance). After six weeks of maintaining that goal weight, they earn a lifetime membership.

NUTRITIONAL EVALUATION   Weight Watchers has kept pretty good pace at integrating the most recent scientific data into its program. The current offering is a high-carbohydrate, reduced-fat, moderate-protein dietary approach. A significant number of Weight Watcher referrals, it should be noted, come from physicians.

The nutrient breakdown of the Weight Watchers diet is as follows:

Carbohydrates 50–60%
Protein 20%
Fat 20–30%
Sodium .... Less than 3,000 milligrams
Fiber .... 20–35 grams

These are the exact pre-1989 U.S. dietary goals. The unlimited vegetables provide good sources of dietary fiber, well within the American Cancer Society's recommendation. A daily-multiple vitamin and mineral supplement is recommended.

Weight Watchers food packages provide very thorough nutritional information—they even break fat content down into the various kinds (helpful for people needing to reduce saturated fat) and provide cholesterol numbers, so that you can easily determine whether a particular Weight Watchers entree is appropriate.

COST   Yearly registration is $32 and includes the first meeting fee. Attendance at weekly meetings is required and costs $11 per week for unlimited meetings that week. Attendance books are stamped at meetings; members missing a week's meetings are required to pay for them. Any member who misses more than a few consecutive meetings, unless for medical or other emergency reasons, must pay $32 to rejoin.

There are no contracts or other long-term financial obligations. There is a significant monetary incentive: members who reach their goal weight and maintain it for six weeks earn lifetime membership allowing them to attend all future meetings for free. Lifetime members must weigh in once a month and, if they regain more than two pounds, must resume paying weekly meeting dues (this is a stringent but often effective rule).

Until maintenance, members may reduce their cost by purchasing prepaid coupons for 10 weeks' worth of meetings at a time and getting two extra weeks' coupons for free. Weight Watchers members may also obtain discounts through participating health maintenance organizations (HMOs); in cases where a physician diagnoses obesity and prescribes Weight Watchers, some insurance companies may provide at least partial reimbursement.

Weight Watchers food products are moderately priced (between $2.00 and $2.50 per entree), but there is no obligation or pressure to buy them, and so the food cost of the program is largely variable.

PRACTICALITY   This is a relatively practical program with no special foods required; everything can be purchased at a supermarket, including Weight Watchers foods. Weight Watchers menus and recipe books are available in bookstores. Traveling members are permitted to attend Weight Watchers meetings at any location.

During the first week of the program, dieters are required to weigh and measure food to determine what the listed quantities look like. They then weigh food once a week to ensure that their judgement has remained accurate. Furthermore, prepackaged Weight Watcher foods are labeled with information directly related to the three levels of the program, eliminating altogether the necessity of weighing.

The Weight Watchers Eating Out & Socializing guide offers tips for staying on the diet at restaurants and parties, with menu ideas for various kinds of ethnic restaurants and plenty of optional calorie (OC) choices. Additional calories are allowed for maximum flexibility and to accommodate special situations. The Healthy Eating guide relates the basic Weight Watcher's guidelines to the goals of reducing intake of saturated fat and cholesterol, excess sugar, and sodium along with increasing complex carbohydrates and fiber. This booklet also addresses moderate alcohol consumption.

For those with lactose intolerance, Weight Watchers claims to have adaptations within its program, but these people must read ingredient labels carefully to ensure they are not putting themselves at risk. Lacto-ovo vegetarians may also use an adaptation of the Weight Watchers program. Weight Watchers even has a special support group for pregnant and lactating women who have obtained the approval of their physicians.

LIFESTYLE AND EXERCISE   Weight Watchers' "Challenges & Choices" booklet focuses on motivation, feelings and stress, social situations, dieting lapses, out-of-control eating, and coping with change. Meetings offer open-group discussion time, called Challenge, to discuss individual problems in losing weight and staying on the diet.

The program is strong on incentives: ribbons and stars are awarded for weight loss accomplishments. All meetings close with celebrations, at which members share their successes.

Exercise is recommended at least 3 times a week with the approval of a physician. Weight Watchers provides an exercise plan booklet, which discusses the benefits of walking, jogging, stationary and outdoor cycling, and swimming. For each listed activity, Weight Watchers provides instructions on stretching, warm-up, execution, cool-down, and safety. These precautions also offer information about exercising at your appropriate activity level and checking your target heart rate, and include a heart rate chart for ease of calculations. Weight Watchers categorizes exercise intensity and duration into four levels, and supplies a questionnaire to help the dieter determine at what level to begin exercising. They also offer specific advice on firming and toning exercises and show how they can be integrated into the dieter's exercise program. Overall, the suggestions are designed for flexibility so as to avoid tedium.

Although the program does not offer its own exercise classes, it gives an award for exercise accomplishments.

WHY IT WORKS   The meetings, which are frequent and conveniently timed, generate a lot of support for members; this support does not end when members reach their goal weight, or even a year or two later. The free lifetime membership for those within two pounds of maintenance weight provides an ongoing support and incentive many people need to keep weight off permanently. Most people who lose weight have to struggle, at least to some degree, the rest of their lives to keep it off; they need continuing support and encouragement.

Weight Watchers teaches weight maintenance skills from the start, enabling dieters to make their own food choices, rather than eat what someone else tells them to. The low cost makes the program available to a large number of people. The variety of the food plan—which includes moderate amounts of pizza, potato chips, cake, ice cream, and chocolate—makes it attractive.

Weight Watchers promotes gradual weight loss and inspires new members with its 30-year reputation and a plethora of success stories from members who have lost weight and kept it off.

POTENTIAL DRAWBACKS   The exercise program suggests but does not require medical supervision. I would, therefore, recommend that anyone with 40 or more pounds to lose seek a doctor's supervision.

While those who run Weight Watchers meetings are trained in the organization's procedures, they are not required to have professional degrees, so those with eating disorders requiring psychological treatment may not find it here. They could, however, follow the program in tandem with professional help.

Finally, since most Weight Watchers members are women, some men may feel uncomfortable in the traditional community groups—although some men may enjoy and be motivated by those demographics.

WEIGHT-CONTROL DIETS

MEDICALLY SUPERVISED DIET PROGRAMS

MEDICALLY SUPERVISED DIET programs are designed primarily for those whose obesity puts them at medical risk, such as diabetics and people with heart disease. A number of these programs require that individuals be at least 20 percent above their ideal body weight before going on a very-low-calorie diet because the larger fat reserves of obese people help to protect their lean muscle tissue from being used by the body as fuel. This is consistent with the 1985 recommendations of the National Institute of Health Consensus Development Panel on the health implications of obesity. The lure of rapid weight loss also attracts many moderately overweight people, but anyone considering this kind of weight loss must consider the many potential health risks.

The various 400–800-calorie-per-day protein-sparing, modified liquid diets usually last about three months, the best of them including a year to 18 months of maintenance. As the name implies, the diet is built around a medically prescribed powdered supplement, often referred to as a "shake." Some programs include one food meal per day in addition to the liquid.

All of these programs are conducted under the supervision of a medical doctor, for good reason. Such rapid weight loss is very stressful on the body in a number of ways and can produce severe side effects.

Very-low-calorie diets (VLCDs), also known as ketogenic diets, put the body in a temporary starvation mode so that the body will burn fat stores, making its primary energy source fat rather than the simple carbohydrate, glucose. That is the desired result. The *un*desired results are numerous. This kind of diet produces excess ketones (substances produced in the liver when it breaks down fat), which stimulate the loss of fluid, sodium, and potassium and can lead to dehydration. These minerals are necessary for heart regularity; in extreme cases, severe deficiencies can lead to coma and death. Medical supervision greatly reduces *but does not altogether eliminate* the risks. A sudden decrease in bodily fluid can create a risk of a sodium/potassium imbalance. This can affect the nervous system, heart rhythm, and other basic cell and body functions.

High complex carbohydrates in VLCDs also help spare body protein, prevent excess fluid loss, and provide increased energy. Some research has indicated that higher-carbohydrate VLCDs may also help keep the patient's metabolic rate from decreasing during the liquid fast.

But even those VLCDs highest in complex carbohydrate are still high in protein and thus are *not recommended for anyone with heart, liver, or kidney problems; anyone with cancer, insulin-dependent diabetes, or psychiatric problems; pregnant women; or the elderly.* Excess protein puts an added stress on key organ function and can exacerbate many existing problems.

On the positive side, the current generation of liquid diets— unlike those of the 1970s, which did not offer high-quality protein sources in their formulas—are, for the most part, nutritionally sound.

Yet they are not without additional risks. Some low-calorie diet programs derive most of their calories from egg white or milk protein. While this may be good-quality protein, using it as a primary source of energy can create a volatile danger for those vulnerable to dietary slips. For someone on such a program, any high-fat binges can produce gastrointestinal distress, since the body's bile acid production will have been greatly reduced by the liquid diet; and the consumption of even moderate amounts of alcohol can lead to severe intoxication, since no bulk foods will be present to help slow the absorption of alcohol into the bloodstream.

Other potential side effects of the very-low-calorie levels can include bad breath, nausea, fatigue, dry skin, hair loss, muscle cramps, sensitivity to cold, and light-headedness. Studies have shown that this kind of severe dieting may also increase an obese person's risk of developing gallstones.

Due to the necessity for close medical supervision, including frequent blood and urine tests and other lab work, and the cost of the prescribed powdered supplement, all VLCDs are—like all other serious medical procedures—expensive.

In weighing the benefit/risk ratio of these diets, consider your chances of success. Recent data show the two-year success rate of all crash diets to be only 2 to 5 percent, and some studies demonstrate a potential disadvantage with liquid diets: comparing dieters who consumed comparable low caloric amounts, the researchers found that those who *ate* rather than just *drank* their calories felt more satisfied and complained less about hunger. This suggests that many people have a need to chew.

Additionally, all rapid-weight-loss diets burn not only fat but also some lean muscle tissue—potentially even the heart muscle; this is very unhealthy and can lead to sudden death. If weight is regained, more fat is taken back on rather than lean muscle tissue. The weight is often regained in the upper body, increasing the risk of heart and other major diseases.

All diets assume some degree of risk; VLCDs assume the most. That is precisely why they are medically supervised and require the recommendation of a physician. Even so, consider the benefit/risk ratio carefully. By being aware of the dangers you can reduce them. You can be on the lookout for the potential adverse side effects and report any to your doctor immediately. VLCDs work—people lose large amounts of weight in a relatively short period of time on them—but they are not for everyone.

HEALTH MANAGEMENT RESOURCES

59 Temple Place, Suite 704
Boston, Massachusetts, 02111
(617) 357-9876

BACKGROUND This company was founded in 1979 by Laurence Stifler, who holds a Ph.D. in experimental psychology from Boston University. The goal is to facilitate safe, rapid weight loss while teaching patients the skills needed to self-manage their weight over a lifetime. HMR has treated more than 200,000 patients in over 600 sites nationwide, located in hospitals, physician group practices, and private medical practices. Staffs vary depending on the size of the program, but each location has at least a medical doctor and a registered nurse. There is a registered dietitian at company headquarters and at some locations.

WHOM IT'S FOR HMR requires that applicants for the core program be at least 20 percent (or at least 30 pounds) over their ideal body weight. There is also a moderately restricted program for anyone with fewer than 30 pounds to lose who is not medically at risk.

HMR screens applicants to determine medical eligibility, and gives an electrocardiogram (EKG) to see whether the individual's condition poses a potential health risk. A physician's referral is recommended but not required.

HOW IT WORKS The program begins with the liquid fast, called the *Weight Loss Phase*, which lasts for a minimum of 12 weeks. Most women are put on the 520-calorie liquid (a powder to which they add water) along with two vitamin and mineral tablets per day. Men are usually given the 800-calorie liquid along with their vitamin/ mineral tablets. HMR also offers an option of using the liquid formula along with solid food for a total of 800 calories per day.

HMR monitors the health of its patients on a weekly basis and performs blood and other lab tests biweekly. Patients get an EKG periodically or at every 25 pounds of weight loss.

The liquid supplements come in a variety of flavors, from chocolate and vanilla to chicken soup. They are more versatile than the formulas of most other liquid diets; they can be mixed cold or heated and can even be used in coffee and other hot beverages. A program recipe booklet provides ways to create additional variations to the listed flavors. Clients are also advised to consume two quarts of liquid per day, including water, coffee, tea, and diet sodas, in addition to the diet supplement.

This fasting phase lasts until the dieter reaches his or her weight goal; the average is about 12 weeks. Dieters attend weekly meetings during which they are weighed, checked by the supervising M.D., consulted by a health educator—sometimes a registered dietitian (with whom the dieter also communicates by phone between in-person consultations)—and are sold the coming week's supply of supplements.

The average weight loss per week is two and a half to five pounds.

The Refeeding Phase lasts from four to six weeks. Each dieter meets weekly with the supervising physician and health educator to discuss and update his or her eating plan. Working together, they create and modify a realistic and workable program. Usually, for the first two weeks of this phase the dieter eats between 500 and 700 calories per day, increasing gradually until the Maintenance phase. Dieters continue to attend classes and communicate by phone with the health educator.

The Maintenance Phase—a requirement—lasts 18 months, during which time calories are individualized according to need. Dieters visit an M.D. weekly, get weighed in, and attend a 60- to 90-minute class with about 15 other maintaining dieters in a closed group. Classes are led by a health educator.

NUTRITIONAL EVALUATION   HMR offers three liquid supplements: a 520-calorie formula for women, an 800-calorie formula for men, and a 520-calorie lactose-free formula for patients with lactose intolerance. Here is how they break down nutritionally:

HMR 500 (for women):

Carbohydrates 60%
Protein 38%
Fat 2%
Sodium . . . . 780 milligrams
Fiber . . . . 4 grams

HMR 800 (for men):
Carbohydrates 49%
Protein 40%
Fat 11%
Sodium . . . . 1,250 milligrams
Fiber . . . . 5 grams

The protein on the 500 and 800 formulas comes from dry non-fat milk and egg white, a high-grade complete protein source, and the carbohydrate is made up of sugars and methycellulose, a good source of fiber—although the fiber level itself is typically low. Daily sodium is acceptable. The protein level for women is adequate (49 grams), but for men it is a bit high (80 grams). Carbohydrates are pleasantly high for the HMR 500. The high-carbohydrate content means that glucose remains a substantial fuel source during weight loss, decreasing the production of ketones with their accompanying negative side effects.

These HMR formulas also provide about 150 percent of the RDAs of most essential vitamins and minerals.

HMR 70 Plus (lactose free):
Carbohydrates 41%
Protein 53%
Fat 6%
Sodium . . . . 920 milligrams
Fiber . . . . 6 grams

HMR 70 Plus gets its protein from egg white solids, a high-grade complete protein source. The carbohydrate level of HMR 70 Plus is about average for this kind of diet; and although sodium levels are good, fiber—as with most VLCDs—is low. Protein is adequate (70 grams)

COST   Prices and rates vary depending on the site; including medical tests, they average approximately $420 per month, with three months the average length of enrollment. Maintenance costs $55 per month. Thus, three months of weight loss and 18 months of maintenance will run about $2,250—anywhere from $40 to $80 per pound lost.

PRACTICALITY   Travel is easier than with most other VLCDs because of program reciprocity: patients may use an HMR site in another city if necessary, or maintain contact with their home-based health educator by phone. The latter alternative makes overseas travel possible.

As with all VLCDs, dining out is tricky at best and frustrating at worst.

LIFESTYLE AND EXERCISE   From the first HMR class, behavior modification is an issue. These mandatory classes last an hour and a half and cover such topics as how to decrease fat, increase exercise, and use the HMR calorie system. Clients are given intensive instruction on the values for all food groups to enable them to make intelligent choices. On maintenance, no food is forbidden—even pizza and beer are allowed. Moderation is stressed.

The meetings also cover exercise strategies, such as ways to increase daily activity. Walking is recommended. Clients study exercise/energy expenditure charts in order to help them visualize ways to burn 2,000 calories each week.

HMR meetings are closed (new dieters must join their own group). Although the group leaders may not be health professionals, they are all trained by HMR.

WHY IT WORKS   HMR offers a liquid diet that can be prepared hot or cold, lessening the potential tedium of such dieting. Their formulas are among the highest in carbohydrates, reducing the possible ketogenic side effects. HMR maintains a national data system to monitor the program's effectiveness and to enhance quality control. Its approach to refeeding and maintenance does not restrict any particular foods, diminishing the chances that the dieter will feel deprived.

According to HMR, the average patient keeps off 60 percent of the initial weight loss after 18- and 24-month follow-ups.

POTENTIAL DRAWBACKS   Because HMR is usually provided in a private physician's office, some locations may not offer the full multidisciplinary approach needed for optimum weight loss and maintenance (though patients can compensate by finding outside sources for exercise and additional group support). Also, the HMR staff often appears to be spread thin. For example, I discovered one HMR dietitian overseeing 30 HMR fasting locations (ideally, each facility should have its own dietitian).

You can guard against both of these drawbacks, however, by making some inquiries and an examination of the particular provider before signing up.

MediBase
2801 Salinas Highway
Building F
Monterey, California, 93940
(800) 553-1754

BACKGROUND MediBase was founded in 1983 in California by Robert Nesheim, who holds a Ph.D. in nutrition from the University of Illinois. Dr. Nesheim is the chairman of the Military Nutrition Committee, a fellow of the American Institute of Nutrition, and has served on the Food and Nutrition Board of the National Academy of Sciences. Today, MediBase is a product of Advanced Healthcare and is available in more than 150 hospitals and private physician practices throughout the United States.

WHOM IT'S FOR MediBase offers two programs. MediBase 420 is for people at least 50 pounds over their ideal body weight *and* have a weight-related medical problem such as diabetes, hypertension, high cholesterol and high triglycerides, or osteoarthritis. MediBase 2 is a more flexible program for people with less weight to lose and no existing medical problem.

HOW IT WORKS MediBase is a one-year program. It begins with a client orientation followed by three distinct phases—*Rapid Weight Loss*, *Transitional Moderate Weight Loss*, and *Maintenance*.

During orientation, each client receives an overview of the program and, with the help of the staff, determines their target weight. In addition, clients are given physical examinations and laboratory tests; each individual is instructed to maintain a food diary which is nutritionally evaluated.

Phase One usually lasts for about twelve weeks and provides a structured program of rapid weight loss. Clients consume three packets per day of MediBase powdered supplement; it is available in chocolate, vanilla, strawberry, and hot chicken soup flavors. MediBase recommends a water intake of three quarts per day in conjunction with this supplement.

Beginning in this phase and continuing through Phase Two, Transition, clients meet with a registered dietitian or (where applicable) a diabetes educator once a week, and a medical doctor for an examination and tests every *other* week.

Additionally, clients meet for individual sessions with counselors and in group classes (usually ten to twelve) to learn about nutrition education, exercise, and other important diet-related subjects. During this phase, the classes emphasize behavioral information, including such topics as the evaluation of peer support needs and the advantages and disadvantages of losing weight.

During Phase Two, the sixteen-week transition period, clients continue to lose weight, though at a moderate rate, as they begin to increase calories. In some cases, solid food is reintroduced. This phase offers two options:

1) Replace the MediBase 420 supplement with the MediBase 2 800-calorie supplement, eventually weaning back onto solid food after achieving goal weight.

2) Remain on MediBase 420 for the first two weeks of Phase Two, reducing the supplement to twice a day. A solid meal is added (which can be either breakfast, lunch, or dinner) for a daily total intake of about 600 calories. Then, for the next two weeks, reduce the supplement to once a day along with *two* solid meals for a daily total of 800 calories. Thereafter, follow a calorie level and meal plan individualized by the client and a registered dietitian.

With either Transition plan, classes with a broader focus still meet once a week. These include important topics about nutrition such as food label reading and reducing dietary fat. Food records are kept and evaluated by a registered dietitian and medical monitoring continues but is reduced to once a month.

Phase Three, Maintenance, lasts for the remainder of the year. During this phase, clients plan and prepare all of their own meals. They are given monthly medical monitoring and attend *bi*weekly classes covering such topics as caffeine consumption, sodium, the role of nutrition in cancer prevention, and food additives. During this period, although the client's diet consists entirely of solid food, MediBase does allow clients to fall back on one powdered supplement per day on hectic or otherwise difficult days.

NUTRITIONAL EVALUATION   MediBase offers two different liquid supplements—a 420-calorie formula for some clients during Phase One and during the transition phase—and the alternative 800-calorie MediBase 2 formula, available for more active clients.

Both formulas get their protein primarily from modified milk whey and soy, and are low in lactose (and therefore, according to a company spokesperson, acceptable for clients with lactose intolerance). Here is how the two MediBase formulas break down nutritionally:

MediBase 420 (three packets per day):
Carbohydrates 51%
Protein 43%
Fat 6%
Sodium .... 1,500 milligrams
Fiber .... 4–6 grams

Though not in line with current recommendations—protein (45 grams) is a bit below the recommended level—carbohydrates do adhere to the pre-1989 levels. Fat and sodium are within acceptable limits. Fiber is low, but MediBase does recommend a fiber supplement for anyone experiencing altered bowel function problems.

MediBase 800 (four packets per day):
Carbohydrates 58%
Protein 25%
Fat 17%
Sodium .... 1,500 milligrams
Fiber .... 5–6 grams

This formula's protein percentage is adequate (50 grams). Carbohydrates, fat, and sodium are well within acceptable limits, but fiber—as with the 420 formula—is low.

COST   The weekly costs—including powdered supplement, counseling, and medical tests—average $63. The full year's program, including maintenance, costs about $3,300. (Prices will vary depending on location.)

PRACTICALITY   The MediBase program requires a minimal number of packets, 3 instead of the usual 5 required in most very-low-calorie liquid diets, thus diminishing the potential fuss of extra mixing. A recipe booklet is provided, with suggestions for varying powdered supplement flavors.

During the first two months of the program, no travel is allowed; class attendance during that time is considered crucial and is therefore mandatory. Later in the program, MediBase permits a one-week vacation, allowing clients to take their powdered supplement on the road.

LIFESTYLE AND EXERCISE   Mandatory classes focus on behavioral modification issues and help dieters break destructive eating habits and become educated eaters so they will be able to maintain their weight loss.

MediBase encourages an exercise regimen beginning—in the fifth week of the program—with walking. The program provides charts and information about activity/caloric expenditures, target heart rate, and group walking. However, like all VLCD programs, MediBase has no formal exercise activity sessions.

WHY IT WORKS   Right from the beginning MediBase offers clients an individualized dieting program. The average weight loss is between two and five pounds per week (2–3 on MediBase 800 and 3–5 on MediBase 420). This is an appropriate rate of **medically-supervised** weight loss, rapid enough to be encouraging to those with a lot to lose.

Group leaders in the meetings are health professionals and the newsletter keeps clients abreast of changes in dieting research findings. The program appears to be relatively flexible in accommodating client needs. Finally, the MediBase 800 formula, among all VLCDs, comes closest to the recommended dietary goals.

POTENTIAL DRAWBACKS   The MediBase program varies between different locations and thus it is not always possible to fully enforce quality control. For example, some group leaders may be better than others and there is no resource for finding this out.

MEDIFAST

11435 Cronhill Drive
P.O. Box 370
Owings Mill, Maryland, 21117-0370
(800) 638-7867

BACKGROUND This program was started by William J. Vitale, M.D., a former Optifast physician. The formula is provided by Jason Pharmaceuticals, Inc., Baltimore. More than 10,000 locations offer the program, mainly in physicians' offices, but also at 120 hospitals on an outpatient basis. Every location has an M.D. on staff; the larger ones also have a registered dietitian and behavioral counselor.

WHOM IT'S FOR Potential patients are not required to have an M.D. referral but must be at least 25 percent above their ideal body weight as determined by the Medifast staff. (A modified program is available for people with less weight to lose.) However, I would *not* recommend any liquid fast without the approval of a personal physician.

HOW IT WORKS This program is built around a natural protein formula enriched with micronutrients in four flavors (strawberry, orange, chocolate, and vanilla). The formula comes in three varieties: Medifast 55 (containing 55 grams of protein) is prescribed for most women; Medifast 70 (70 grams of protein), used by most men on the program, is higher in protein and lower in carbohydrates. Medifast Plus (98 grams of protein), to be taken along with one food meal per day, is for men or women who are only 20 to 30 pounds above their ideal body weight, or who have physically demanding jobs that would make any potential light-headedness dangerous.

The four-phase program lasts 42 weeks.

Orientation lasts for approximately one week. During this phase, patients undergo a medical evaluation, including an EKG, blood and urine analysis, blood pressure reading, weigh-in, and computerized body-fat analysis. They learn what to expect from the program and fill out necessary paperwork.

Weight Reduction lasts until the dieter reaches his or her ideal weight. The length varies according to the doctor's individual recommendation; the average is 16 weeks. During this phase, the client consumes five powdered supplements per day at a calorie level of 450. All Medifast supplements must be mixed with eight ounces of liquid: water, mineral water, club soda, or sugar-free drinks. (There is a modified Medifast 55 program—for men as well as women— which allows the five supplements plus one meal, bringing the daily calories to 800; according to Medifast, the additional meal does not appear to slow down the rate of weight loss among most of its clients.)

Refeeding (also referred to as realimentation) lasts from four to six weeks and gradually reintroduces solid foods, reducing the powdered supplement. A sample refeeding schedule might look like this:

Week one—Each day, four packets of powdered supplement, four ounces of lean protein, and one-half cup of cooked vegetables.

Week two—Add one fruit.

Week three—Reduce powdered supplement to three packets per day; add two more ounces of lean protein, one cup of salad vegetables, and a cup of nonfat milk.

Week four—Add two servings of bread or cereals.

Week five—Reduce powdered supplement to two packets per day; increase nonfat milk to two cups, and add another serving of fresh fruit.

Week six—Eliminate supplement completely; add two more bread or cereal servings.

Where appropriate, supervising physicians allow dietary modifications for vegetarian clients or those with specific food preferences or allergies. An extra packet of powdered supplement is often prescribed for clients experiencing light-headedness.

Maintenance lasts 12 weeks. At this point, the client's diet is individualized to maintain his or her ideal weight.

Throughout the program, there is an emphasis on one-on-one counseling, since most Medifast programs are run out of private physicians' offices. Some larger programs may also provide group meetings led by a health professional. Patients meet biweekly with the supervising doctor and are weighed and examined weekly.

According to Medifast, typical weight loss is between 3.6 and 5.2 pounds per week.

NUTRITIONAL EVALUATION   The 840 calories for men and the 450 or 800 calories for women break down as follows:

Medifast 55 (five packets total 450 calories):
Carbohydrates 41%
Protein 50%
Fat 9%
Sodium . . . . 930 milligrams
Fiber . . . . 6 grams

The daily fiber intake is very low. I would recommend about 20 to 30 grams; the deficiency could alter bowel function. Sodium levels are well within the U.S. dietary goals. Because of the low caloric levels, vitamin and mineral supplementation is part of the program, to bring it up to 100 percent or more of each nutrient's USRDA.

Medifast 70 (five packets total 800 calories):
Carbohydrates 38%
Protein 59%
Fat 3%
Sodium . . . . 920 milligrams
Fiber . . . . 2 grams

As with Medifast 55, fiber is low but the sodium level is good. Supplementation provides good vitamin and mineral content. The protein level is very high (118 grams).

Medifast Plus (four packets total 390 calories; not including the additional 450-calorie meal per day):
Carbohydrates 59%
Protein 35%
Fat 6%
Sodium . . . . 468 milligrams
Fiber . . . . 3 grams

Because this powdered supplement is higher in carbohydrates, the risk of ketone production and lean muscle tissue loss is significantly reduced. Protein is satisfactory (73 grams). Otherwise, it meets the same health guidelines as Medifast's other formulas.

COST   Medifast locations charge $65–$85 per week, which brings the total program cost to about $3,000. This does not include the cost of blood tests. According to Medifast, most insurance companies will cover office visits and medical tests.

LIFESTYLE AND EXERCISE   Medifast offers weekly one-hour classes led by a registered dietitian, and a monthly open forum led by a behavioral psychologist. The weekly lifestyle classes address such issues as self-esteem, assertiveness, compulsiveness, restaurant dining, low-fat cooking demonstrations, how to read nutritional labels, and stress management. Regular attendance is emphasized but not mandatory, and cassette tapes are available covering nutrition and exercise as well as behavioral modification.

The behavioral modification program is divided into two phases. During *Lifestyles 1* (weeks 1–21), clients learn behavioral modification techniques. During *Lifestyles 2* (weeks 22–42, running concurrently with the maintenance phase of the diet), clients learn to apply those skills in real-life situations—more of a hands-on approach, including cooking demonstrations. Unfortunately, not all Medifast locations offer the Lifestyles 2 program, so you may want to inquire before signing on at a particular location.

The Medifast program encourages exercise, recommending a brisk walk (one mile at 3.5 mph or greater, with gradual increases) as the best transitional activity for the recently sedentary. Some larger Medifast sites may have an exercise physiologist to monitor exercise rates; at other sites the supervising physician performs that service.

PRACTICALITY   As with all very-low-calorie diet programs, restrictions and inconveniences are inherent—travel is discouraged and dining out is difficult. Medifast does provide a recipe guide for flavor variation with the powdered supplements, and a hot supplement soup which provides the same nutritional value as the cold supplement drinks may also be used. In addition, the Medifast formula is available for sale directly to doctors, so the program need not be hospital based.

WHY IT WORKS   The counseling staff is professional and well-trained and pays close attention to the client's needs. This seems to help mitigate the frustration and hopelessness that often accom-

pany attempts to lose large amounts of weight. The powdered supplements come in a variety of flavors, are easy to prepare, and
eliminate the anxiety of deciding what to eat. According to Medifast, 65 percent of the clients who finish the program remain within
four pounds of their ideal weight during the first year thereafter.

POTENTIAL DRAWBACKS   Aside from the drawbacks basic to
all VLCDs, Medifast, because it is offered mostly through private
medical practices, provides only minimal support staff. This may
hinder the program's ability to present the multidisciplinary approach recommended for this kind of diet. Medifast does not, for
example, require nutritional counseling or support groups except
where it is offered in a hospital setting. The organization claims,
however, to have begun to require Medifast sites to provide such
services.

OPTIFAST

5320 W. 23rd Street
Minneapolis, Minnesota 55440
(800) 328-5392

BACKGROUND   Optifast was begun in 1976 by Sandoz Nutrition and was the first program of this kind. Today the Optifast program is offered at 600 centers nationwide, including Optifast clinics, participating hospitals (on an outpatient basis), and private group physician practices.

Along with being the oldest medically supervised weight loss program, Optifast is also among the most successful, especially since its highly promoted association with television star Oprah Winfrey and her 67-pound weight loss (much of which she subsequently regained).

WHOM IT'S FOR   To be eligible for this 26-week program, the individual must be referred by a physician and be 30 percent above ideal body weight and at least 50 pounds overweight, or 20 percent above ideal body weight and at medical risk. Anyone with less than 50 pounds to lose would risk losing lean muscle tissue. (Like Medifast, Optifast also has modified programs for individuals with less weight to lose.)

All patients must submit to an EKG before being admitted to ensure that they are not at risk for heart failure.

HOW IT WORKS   The first week of the program is an orientation period. Each dieter helps provide a medical and psychological history, is given an overview of what is ahead, and is then assigned to a group.

The diet itself begins with the *Modified Fast*, a medically supervised, low-calorie, high-protein liquid diet. Women are usually given Optifast 70 (420 calories per day and lactose free), while men are prescribed Optifast 800 (800 calories per day). These 80-calorie liquid supplements come in the form of a flavored (orange, cherry, chocolate, or vanilla), high-quality protein powder, enriched with vitamins and minerals. It is mixed with a noncaloric beverage.

According to Optifast, approximate weight loss is three to five pounds (or 1–2 percent of the client's body weight) per week. If a patient is losing weight at an unhealthfully rapid rate, the supervising physician can mediate by raising caloric intake accordingly.

The Modified Fast phase lasts for only 12 weeks even if the client has not reached his or her goal weight—this in accordance with clinical studies showing 12 weeks as the maximum time anyone should be on such a regimen. Optifast has also found that this structure reduces the patient dropout rate. All patients are given another EKG before entering the next phase of the program.

In *Realimentation* (also known as refeeding), a six-week phase, the liquid diet is gradually reduced as solid food is increased. A sample daily refeeding schedule might look like this:

Week one—Each day, four packets of powdered supplement, four ounces of lean meat (beef, fish, or poultry), and one-half cup cooked vegetables, such as broccoli, carrots, or green beans.

Week two—Same as above plus one fresh fruit per day.

Week three—Decrease to three packets of powdered supplement; add two additional ounces protein, one cup nonfat milk, and one cup salad.

Week four—Add two servings from the bread/cereal group.

Week five—Decrease to two packets of powdered supplement; add one raw and two cooked vegetables and two fresh fruits.

Week six—Decrease to one packet of powdered supplement; add two servings of bread or cereal and one more cup of nonfat milk.

By the end of Realimentation, the powdered supplement has been completely eliminated and the dieter eats three meals per day based upon an individualized plan created with the help of a registered dietitian. For women, this plan usually contains 1,200–1,500 calories per day; for men, 1,500–1,800. The meal plan can be altered to accommodate vegetarians or those with specific food allergies or preferences.

For the next seven weeks, during *Stabilization*, clients follow these food plans and exercise to maintain their weight loss. At the end of the 26th week, clients are given another EKG.

During all phases of Optifast, clients must drink one to two quarts of water per day to flush out the ketones produced when the body changes its primary fuel source from glucose to fat. This increased fluid consumption also helps to maintain the body's electrolyte balance. Throughout the program, clients are given periodic medical examinations, including blood tests and urinalyses to ensure good health and a minimum of side effects. For at least the first 21 weeks, clients are weighed weekly by a registered nurse and given nutritional counseling by a registered dietitian.

Weekly group support meetings bring together 15 to 20 clients and a health professional (for example, a behaviorist, an exercise physiologist, or a registered dietitian). These group leaders review food and exercise diaries and discuss specific problem-solving techniques. The group support meetings are mandatory; failure to attend may lead to expulsion from the program.

The *Encore* maintenance phase of Optifast is an optional extra period of support group meetings—7 weekly meetings and 26 biweekly meetings, 60 to 90 minutes long.

NUTRITIONAL EVALUATION   The caloric levels (420 for women, 800 for men) are broken down as follows:

Optifast 70:
Carbohydrates 29%
Protein 67%
Fat 4%
Sodium .... 900 milligrams
Fiber 0

Optifast 800:
Carbohydrates 50%
Protein 35%
Fat 15%
Sodium .... 1,150 milligrams
Fiber 0

Although the caloric percentages differ, the actual amount of protein is about the same (70 grams) in both powdered supplements. The higher fat percentage in Optifast 800 is due, in part, to the presence of increased soybean oil.

The sodium content conforms to U.S. dietary goals, and while neither drink contains fiber, Optifast offers a psyllium-based fiber supplement (three grams of fiber per packet). The use of this fiber supplement should lessen the possibility of bowel irregularity. The supervising physician prescribes the correct amount for the individual.

Enriched with vitamins and minerals, the powdered supplement meets or exceeds 100% of all the USRDAs.

COST   Optifast charges approximately $500 per month. A six-month program, including the powdered meals, costs approximately $2,800–$3,200 (varying by location). That comes to between $40 and $70 per pound. The Encore maintenance costs approximately $300–$400, or about $15–$20 per session. If the referring M.D. provides a written prescription for weight loss, some insurance programs may cover a portion of the Optifast cost.

PRACTICALITY   Optifast requires a large investment of time—the weekly sessions, weigh-ins, medical tests, and other supervision can add up. Since special diet products are an integral part of this program and medical supervision is essential, eating out and traveling are limited. In fact, clients are advised not to travel for longer than one week and may do so only with the supervising physician's and the program's consent. At present, there are no arrangements for traveling patients to use centers other than the one they are enrolled in (although centers will transfer patients relocating on a permanent basis).

Naturally, Optifast dieters responsible for feeding other family members will have the added work of preparing separate meals.

LIFESTYLE AND EXERCISE   Weekly behavior modification meetings begin in the first week and last through the 26th. Group leaders are behavioral counselors, registered dietitians, or exercise physiologists. Topics of discussion include eating in social situations, structured meal planning, conditioned hunger, lapses (small set-backs) and relapses (complete dropping of diet for an extended period), and how to get back on track. Group support meeting attendance is mandatory.

Exercise is encouraged throughout the program in the group discussions. An exercise physiologist prescribes an individualized exercise program for each client, provides an exercise diary, and reviews it every week with the client, giving advice on techniques to develop a more active lifestyle.

WHY IT WORKS   Optifast works for much the same reasons as Medifast—fast results can be encouraging.

As for its success rate, the largest study of Optifast was conducted in 1988 at Kaiser Permanente Medical Center in San Diego. Of 2,200 clients, 55 percent dropped out of the program and regained most of their lost weight. While this may sound high, it probably isn't. In fact, Optifast is the only VLCD program that has published any such data to date. This suggests that they are at least average—and possibly above average—in success for this kind of diet. Furthermore, Optifast executives claim that program improvements have reduced the dropout rate to about 40%.

POTENTIAL DRAWBACKS   Not all Optifast locations provide exactly the same program. Some may offer a stronger behavioral modification component and weight maintenance program than others. Twenty-six weeks is not a lot of time in which to change destructive eating habits—especially when the first 12 weeks are a liquid fast. These drawbacks, however, are relatively minor in relation to the potential problems associated with all diets of this category.

Optitrim

5320 W. 23rd Street

Minneapolis, Minnesota 55440

(800) 328-5392

BACKGROUND   This is a recent offshoot of the Optifast program, designed to accommodate the need for a modified medically supervised weight loss program that does not require total dependence on a liquid fast. There are 300 hospital-affiliated centers providing Optitrim.

WHOM IT'S FOR   The Optitrim program is for people who need to lose more than 20 but less than 50 pounds or who are 20 percent above their ideal body weight, but do not face an immediate medical risk.

Optitrim does not *require* a physician's referral, but potential clients are screened with a medical/behavioral questionnaire along with a medical exam, which includes a blood chemistry analysis.

HOW IT WORKS   During the first eight weeks of the Optitrim program, called *Phase One*, dieters eat 975 calories per day, consisting of the powdered supplement (added to water to make a shake) three times a day and one Opti Entree, a prepackaged meal of solid food. Weekly behavioral modification classes begin during Phase One and continue throughout the duration of the program. Once a week, clients are also weighed and given a medical check-up, including a blood pressure reading. After the first four weeks, a blood chemistry analysis is repeated.

For the next six weeks of Optitrim, called the *Transition Phase*, caloric intake is increased to 1,100–1,200 calories per day. This is a refeeding period—a transition back to a diet entirely of solid food. The process goes as follows:

Weeks 9–11: two servings per day of powdered supplement, one Opti Entree and one self-prepared meal.

Weeks 12–14: one serving per day of powdered supplement, one Opti Entree, one self-prepared dinner, and a self-prepared snack.

Sometime between weeks 13 and 15 the client meets with a registered dietitian to individualize a meal plan for maintenance.

The *Optitrim Maintenance Phase* lasts four weeks. The dieter consumes between 1,200 and 2,000 calories per day of self-prepared meals. This caloric level—which can, in some cases, even exceed 2,000—is determined by sex, height, frame-size, and activity level.

In addition to the Maintenance Phase of the program, Optitrim also offers a 6-month *Encore Maintenance* program, the same one offered in the Optifast program.

NUTRITIONAL EVALUATION   The 975 calories per day during Phase One (consisting of three powdered supplements along with one Opti Entree) break down as follows:

Carbohydrates 50%
Protein 28%
Fat 22%
Sodium . . . . 1,650 milligrams
Fiber . . . . a minimum of 5 grams

The 1,100 to 1,200 calories per day during Phase Two (three powdered supplements, one Opti Entree plus one self-prepared meal) break down as follows:

Carbohydrates 50–55%
Protein 25–28%
Fat 20–24%
Sodium . . . . 1,500–1,700 milligrams
Fiber . . . . a minimum of 5 grams

The protein percentages are higher than those recommended in the U.S. dietary goals, but the gram levels are reasonable. Since the calories are low, it might otherwise be difficult to get adequate protein intake. Carbohydrates adhere to pre-1989 recommended levels. Fat and sodium are well within acceptable limits. Fiber, however, is low—though more so during Phase One than in Phase Two.

COST   Depending on the location, 18 weeks of the Optitrim program can cost anywhere from $1,300 to $1,800.

PRACTICALITY   Like any medically supervised diet, Optitrim requires a substantial investment of time. However, since the Opti

Entrees are shelf-stable, dieter's can enjoy some freedom to travel—
though extended travel is discouraged.

LIFESTYLE AND EXERCISE   Like Optifast, behavior modification
meetings are a substantial part of this weight-loss program. Class
size is about fifteen people. These meetings are closed to new dieters, who are assigned to their own groups. Group-support meeting
attendance is mandatory.

Optitrim encourages a walking program approved by an M.D.
Exercise begins during the fourth week of the program and is approached in a gradual manner, enabling the dieter slow and realistic
increases in frequency, intensity, and duration of physical activity.

WHY IT WORKS   Optitrim works for many of the same reasons
as Optifast, with the increased benefits of the Opti Entrees and self-
prepared meals. The diet is still very low in calories, but being able
to chew food has been shown to improve dieter satisfaction and
thus may contribute to successful weight loss. The opportunity to
select and prepare one's own meals after 8 weeks can only enhance
the dieter's chances of long-term success in maintaining weight loss.

POTENTIAL DRAWBACKS   Optitrim offers 4 weeks of maintenance as a part of the core program. While the more significant
6 month maintenance program is only treated as optional, it should
be mandatory. For most overweight people to be successful at weight
control, maintenance is not an option—it's a necessity.

United Weight Control Corporation

425 West 59th Street, Suite 5C
New York, New York, 10019
(212) 956-8922

BACKGROUND This program was founded in 1986 by Theodore Van Itallie, M.D., who conducted the primary research at St. Luke's Roosevelt Hospital in New York City. At present there are five locations—two in New York City, one on Long Island, one in Philadelphia, and one in Boston. The focus of the program is on what is termed "individual quality weight loss," which is another way of saying they want their clients to lose fat and not lean muscle tissue. United offers three variations of its program: the Permanence Program, the Modified Permanence Program, and the Risk Reduction Program. They differ primarily in caloric composition and in terms of what kind of obesity they are designed to reverse.

WHOM IT'S FOR Dieters must have a body mass index greater than 28 (lower if you have a medical problem associated with obesity). Body mass index (BMI) is a metric method of computing a person's height/weight ratio in order to determine obesity. Those patients with less weight to lose may elect to go on the Modified Permanence Program, a combination of solid foods and liquid formula with an emphasis on individualization of diet. United's Risk Reduction Program is specialized for patients (usually men) with predominantly upper-body obesity. To qualify for this program, also a combination of solid foods and liquid formula, clients must have a waist-to-hip ratio of one or more (meaning that the waist is as large as or larger than the hips).

HOW IT WORKS The *Beginning Phase* lasts 13 weeks. The first week consists of medical testing, including an EKG and a body composition examination that measures fat (which is what you want to lose) and lean body tissue (which you don't want to lose). This test is subsequently repeated every two months so that the supervising health-care professional can make the necessary adjustments to ensure the minimum loss of lean body mass. The second and third weeks consist of orientation. They are followed by 10 weeks of liquid fasting on a formula of 600–1,400 calories per day (individualized for each client). During this phase, United provides weekly one-hour nutrition education classes taught by a registered dietitian. Clients are examined by the supervising physician and blood tests are run on alternating weeks.

After 10 weeks on the liquid fast, those clients who have reached their ideal body weight move on to the Refeeding Phase. Those who have not yet reached their goal enter the Advanced Phase.

During the *Advanced Phase*, nutrition classes are more advanced. Otherwise, it is an extension of the first 10 weeks and continues until the client reaches his or her goal weight; on the average this phase lasts about 10 weeks.

The *Refeeding Phase* lasts 4 to 8 weeks and gradually reintroduces solid food into the diet. A typical 1,000-calorie example:

Week one—600 calories from formula, 400 from food

Week two—400 calories from formula, 600 from food

Week three—200 calories from formula, 800 from food

Week four—No formula, 1,000 calories from food

The *Maintenance Phase* lasts for at least one year. Food and exercise diaries are maintained and program participants practice nutritional strategies taught in earlier classes.

NUTRITIONAL EVALUATION   This is where the three varieties of United's program differ most.

Permanence Program (liquid diet):
Carbohydrates 48%
Protein 46%
Fat 6%
Sodium . . . . 880 milligrams
Fiber . . . . 6 grams

The carbohydrate percentage is probably adequate to help prevent ketosis, but protein is very high (115 grams). Sodium and fat levels are within a safe range; fiber, as expected, is low.

Modified Permanence Program (liquid diet with some meals):
Carbohydrates 57%
Protein 33%
Fat 10%
Sodium .... 1,300 to 1,400 milligrams
Fiber .... approx. 6 grams or more

The high percentage of carbohydrates makes ketone formation extremely unlikely. Sodium is higher than most VLCDs due to the inclusion of solid food, but still within acceptable health guidelines. Fiber is surprisingly low, considering that solid food is a part of the diet. Protein is only slightly high (83 grams).

Risk Reduction Program (for upper-body obesity):
Carbohydrates 69%
Protein 28%
Fat 3%
Sodium .... 1,000 milligrams
Fiber .... 11 grams

Ketones should not be a problem with this diet since the primary fuel source remains glucose due to the higher level of carbohydrates. Sodium is reasonable but fiber is low. Dieters must be sure to include adequate water and fiber intake to ensure proper bowel function. Protein is at a good level (70 grams).

COST   At an average of $665 per month (including formula and medical testing), the cost for a 40-pound weight loss is about $1,995, or about $50 per pound.

PRACTICALITY   United is neither much more nor less practical than most other very-low-calorie diets. Travel is limited to one week with a doctor's approval; dining out, though not impossible, can be difficult.

LIFESTYLE AND EXERCISE   United provides weekly classes led by a registered dietitian. Topics include dietary fat, cholesterol, and calorie counting. Program staff continually monitor clients in order to make necessary adjustments. Each location has either an occupational therapist or exercise physiologist to help clients customize and then monitor an exercise program.

WHY IT WORKS   United performs body composition testing, using an electromagnetic scanner to measure the ratio of fat to lean muscle mass. This is one of the most accurate predictors of fat loss. United is, to my knowledge, the only VLCD using this technology. Also, maintenance is relatively inexpensive ($550 for a year) and United offers a maintenance rebate for anyone who stays on maintenance for at least six months—giving an extra financial incentive not only to lose the weight but to keep it off.

Since this is not a franchised organization, United offers greater quality control and consistency over the services provided. United's sites are all affiliated with teaching hospitals that, according to a company spokesperson, "take obesity very seriously and keep the program on its toes."

United's Risk Reduction Program is the only one of its kind and can be effective for the particular needs of obese men.

POTENTIAL DRAWBACKS   The drawbacks are no different from those of most other VLCDs. Patients can encounter bowel irregularities and the dissatisfaction of not having food to chew that is associated with liquid diets.

WEIGH TO LIVE

2311 205th Street, Suite 103
Torrance, California, 90501

(800) 554-LIVE

BACKGROUND   This plan was developed by George A Bray, M.D. According to a company spokesperson, it began in 1982. There are eight centers in four states (New York, New Jersey, California, and Hawaii), all franchised to hospitals. All staff are health professionals (physicians, registered dietitians, or behavior counselors) who are trained by the organization in the program philosophy.

WHOM IT'S FOR   Patients must be 25 percent above ideal body weight, or 20 percent above and at medical risk. Weigh to Live requires a physician's referral.

HOW IT WORKS   The first phase, *Weight Control*, lasts for 16 weeks or until the client reaches his or her goal weight. During this phase, the dieter may choose from one of three program variations:

1. A liquid formula of 650–800 calories. This powdered supplement comes in chocolate and vanilla and is served cold. The amounts are individualized to suit the dieter's needs.

2. The Menu Max Plan, which uses food purchased by the client at a supermarket. Customized to the dieter by an on-site registered dietitian, this diet emphasizes foods with the highest nutrient density (the most nutrients per calorie).

3. A combination of the above—a computer program calculates caloric equivalents between regular food and the liquid formula, enabling the dieter to decide which to consume at any given meal.

The Weight Control phase is followed by four weeks of *Maintenance*, at which time the dieter is given an individualized meal program that may include some of the liquid formula. It aims to establish a calorie level that will stabilize weight at the new level.

The last phase of Weigh to Live is *Access*, an ongoing, lifelong program for continued support after the achievement of ideal body weight.

NUTRITIONAL EVALUATION   Weigh to Live offers two different formulas, which provide calories as follows:

Formula 650:
Carbohydrates 40%
Protein 42%
Fat 18%
Sodium .... 1,000 milligrams
Fiber 0*

Formula 800:
Carbohydrates 56%
Protein 30%
Fat 14%
Sodium .... 1,000 milligrams
Fiber 0*

The carbohydrate percentage would seem to be adequate to significantly reduce ketones and protein is adequate to help preserve lean muscle mass. Sodium and fat levels are both acceptable.

COST   Cost of the liquid diet program ranges from $400 to $450 depending on location; this includes all medical tests, powdered formula, and four to six weeks of Maintenance. This comes to as little as $10 per pound—the least expensive of the VLCDs reviewed here. For an additional $20 per month members may continue to attend biweekly maintenance classes, and attend additional classes if desired for $10 each.

The cost of the Menu Max program ranges from $79 to $99, depending on the clinic, and includes medical tests, weigh-ins, and nutritional and other guidance. Since this plan allows the client to purchase his or her own food from the market, the total cost will vary. Lifetime maintenance is, as above, $20 per month for biweekly classes, plus $10 per extra class.

---

*Fiber supplements are left up to the client and supervising physician or dietitian; doctors sometimes prescribe Metamucil.

Weigh to Live's combination plan varies in cost depending upon the ratio of formula to regular food consumed. Costs for lifetime maintenance are the same as above.

PRACTICALITY   This program is different from other hospital-based programs in that the dieter can choose which of the three variations is best suited to his or her needs. Since one of the plans lets the dieter eat real food rather than rely on a liquid supplement, this makes travel and dining out much easier than with other very-low-calorie diets, although medical supervision does create some restrictions. The program's menu variations are designed to accommodate those who follow kosher or vegetarian diets, or who are lactose- or gluten-intolerant.

LIFESTYLE AND EXERCISE   There are weekly meetings, both one-on-one and group support. Anyone can join the support groups at any time.

Four weeks into the diet, the supervising doctor or dietitian provides each client with an individualized exercise program to facilitate a transition from what is usually a sedentary life to a lifestyle that includes such activities as brisk walking, stationary bike riding, and swimming. Activity levels are monitored by the supervising physician. Each patient is encouraged to keep an exercise diary along with a food diary.

WHY IT WORKS   Weigh to Live's Formula 800 is high in carbohydrates, reducing the risk of ketones and other potential VLCD side effects. Also, this program offers choices that enable the dieter to begin to take control from the start. The lifelong support of the *Access* feature is something all diet programs should have. Weight control *is* a lifelong issue.

POTENTIAL DRAWBACKS   Weigh to Live has many of the same risks as any other very-low-calorie diet. Additionally, the open-meeting format of the behavioral modification program can reduce the support, bonding, and confidence more easily established in closed-group sessions. But probably the most significant negative feature of Weigh to Live is location. With only eight sites, it is simply not available to most people.

WEIGHT-CONTROL DIETS

WEIGHT-LOSS BOOKS

OF ALL THE AVAILABLE WEIGHT loss plans, diet books are by far the most plentiful, and therefore the most difficult category from which to make a limited selection. I have tried here to present worthwhile examples from a variety of different approaches to weight loss. Some are complete programs addressing food, behavior, and exercise. Others address only one or two of those components but do so in an effective way and can thus become part of successful weight control.

I tried to represent the best of not only the more popular and well-known diet books of recent years but also the best of some lesser-known but equally worthy books. Obviously, these do not represent the *only* good diet books, but they do represent a wide spectrum of points of view from doctors, nutritionists, dietitians, as well as lay people who draw from research and their own personal experience with weight control. Think of these books as a collection from which you can confidently make a selection based not only upon the features of the diet but also upon the authority of the author.

Beginning in this section and for the remainder of this book, the format of the listings will change somewhat. Unlike diet programs, diet books are not predetermined courses of action. Though some prescribe very specific recommendations, including menu plans and recipes, the implementation of the diet is nevertheless left entirely to the dieter. Thus, the heading *How it works* no longer fits; how a diet book works is entirely dependent on the reader. This heading will be replaced with the more appropriate *Overview*.

The *Nutritional evaluation* portion of most diets in this section will include, in addition to the carbohydrate/protein/fat breakdown and the sodium and fiber content, cholesterol count and a bar graph calculating how well a typical day's menu meets the recommended daily requirements for a range of important nutrients. Although you can take supplements to compensate for any shortfall in the diet, nutrients are almost always best absorbed and utilized when they come from food sources.

In the bar chart, the initials RA/RM denote daily Recommended Allowance and Recommended Maximum.

In order to give the most accurate reading, the results, wherever possible, reflect an average of two days' menu plans. The standards against which these diets are measured come from a variety of sources: *Calories; protein; iron; calcium; phosphorus; Vitamins A, B-1 (thiamin), B-2 (riboflavin), C, B-6 and B-12; zinc; niacin,* and *folacin* are based on the recommended dietary allowances established by the National Academy of Sciences in 1989. (Note: Some calorie-restricted diets specifically list the number of calories. Where they have not, the analysis has included the recommended calories for the hypothetical dieter.)

The *cholesterol* standard is based on the American Heart Association recommendations. The *carbohydrate* and *fat-from-calories* standards are based on the U.S. Dietary Goals, and the *fiber* standard comes from the National Cancer Institute.

The *sodium* maximum is from the Food and Nutrition Board's "Diet and Health," while the *potassium* recommendation is from the "Estimated Minimum Requirements for Healthy Persons," RDA, 1989.

For example: If a bar chart shows Protein at 200 percent and Calcium at 50 percent, it means that the particular diet being discussed provides twice the recommended amount of protein and one-half the recommended amount of calcium. In some cases, too much or too little of a nutrient can contribute to health problems, but this is not much to be concerned about for people who are eating more than 1,000 calories a day, and are consuming a balance of foods and nutrients. Again, remember that many of these books were published before the revised 1989 guide-lines for RDAs; also bear in mind that in many diets, some nutrients are less than 100 percent of the RDA but above two-thirds of those guidelines. Two-thirds of the RDA, while not ideal, is nevertheless safe and will not, according to the National Academy of Sciences, lead to nutritional deficiencies.

Since nutritional needs vary depending on age and gender, it was necessary to select a hypothetical person—in most cases 35-year-old female—in order to make accurate ratings. The conclusions are, nevertheless, fairly universal since the same RDAs would apply to healthy adults between the ages of 25 and 50, and there is little gender distinction.

The nutritional analyses were prepared by Computrition, Inc. (Chatsworth, California), a highly respected computerized nutritional analysis company with the most extensive food database of more than 17,000 food items. Their clients include the University of California at Los Angeles, the American Dietetic Association's National Center for Nutrition and Dietetics, *Cooking Light* magazine, the United States Marine Corps and the United States Olympic Training Center.

One bit of insight you won't need spelled out for you in the coming sections of this book is cost. Everyone knows the approximate cost of a book, and the cost of the food recommended in any text isn't likely to exceed what you would normally purchase (in fact, it's often *cheaper* than what you've been eating).

I am not the first to evaluate these diet books. You should know what others have said as well, and so I have added the heading *Second opinion* (some also contain a third opinion). While most of these other viewpoints do not contradict my assessments, they nevertheless shed additional insight. Many of these review excerpts come from *Current Diet Review* and *Environmental Nutrition Newsletter*, journals for dietitians and other health professionals. A number of review excerpts were also taken from *Publishers Weekly*, a trade periodical for the book industry, and *Library Journal*, a trade periodical for libraries.

Although most people with weight problems suffer from being overweight, there are also those in search of safe and effective ways to put pounds on. With them in mind, this section will end with advice on how to modify weight loss diets for healthful weight gain.

One final word about diet books: They require on the part of the reader a great amount of self-imposed structure, discipline, and motivation. This is beneficial for some people but detrimental for others. The best advice on that issue is: *Be honest with yourself about your limitations, but don't underestimate your potential for change.*

THE CHOOSE TO LOSE DIET: A FOOD LOVER'S GUIDE TO PERMANENT WEIGHT LOSS

by Ron Goor, Ph.D., Nancy Goor, and
Katherine Boyd, R.D.
Houghton Mifflin Company
Boston: 1990

ABOUT THE AUTHORS   Ron Goor holds a doctorate in biochemistry as well as a master's in public health from Harvard University. He is director of Health Prospects, a division of Prospect Associates, a biomedical consulting firm whose primary client is the National Institute of Health. He helps develop programs and educational materials about cholesterol and heart disease.

Nancy Goor is a writer and cook. Katherine Boyd is a senior nutritionist at Health Prospects.

The three are also authors of the best-selling *Eater's Choice: A Food Lover's Guide to Lower Cholesterol.*

WHOM IT'S FOR   As the title suggests, this book is aimed at people who enjoy eating and don't want to completely sacrifice this pleasure in order to lose weight and keep it off.

OVERVIEW   This book focuses on dietary fat reduction as the single most important factor in weight loss. It details a diet built around complex carbohydrates with adequate protein and very low fat, coupled with an exercise program to ensure that the body burns fat rather than lean muscle tissue.

The Choose to Lose program begins with recommendations about determining the correct caloric intake to achieve ideal body weight. The first step is for dieters to keep a three-day food diary for the purpose of determining the fat content of the foods they habitually eat. Next, dieters use a worksheet to help make calculations along with desired-weight tables that take into account body frame size. The authors correctly urge that no one should go on a diet of fewer than 1,000 calories per day.

Although dieters are advised to set total caloric intake levels, fat percentage is emphasized even more. The authors list three fat budget levels: 20 percent, 17 percent, and 15 percent of daily calories from fat. They recommend starting at 20 percent, maintaining that for three to four weeks, then lowering it with the eventual goal of 15 percent. The authors use the word *budget* to underscore the idea that weight control is a matter of choices. If you are allotted 15 or 20 percent of your daily calories as fat, no foods are absolutely restricted, but it's understood that if you choose to eat a double fudge brownie, this may comprise half your entire day's fat allotment in about three bites—much the same way that one shopping spree can use up your entire monthly spending budget.

As with a financial budget, it is necessary to keep records. The authors suggest a food diary of calorie and fat consumption in order to ensure adherence to the diet as well as an awareness of food choices and their ramifications—and they stress honesty.

The book devotes a good deal of space to the realities of fat in common foods, shattering the myth of the typical "dieter's plate"— the bunless hamburger with cottage cheese—which may be low in calories but is often high in fat and thus does not facilitate weight loss. The book also gives practical guidelines for identifying visible and invisible fat and avoiding both kinds.

There are recipes for low-fat versions of high-fat foods such as pizza, along with advice for avoiding dietary fat in such situations as fast-food eating (which the authors deplore but accept as an occasional necessity), snacks, and desserts. They point out that dietary sugar is not the cause of obesity—the sweets that put on pounds are the ones high in fat, such as cookies and donuts. Hard candies, jellies, jams, and syrups are, according to the authors, sound alternatives to chocolates and butter. They recommend no-fat snacks such as pretzels rather than high-fat chips.

Choose to Lose suggests planning your meals and shows how a typical working woman can do so. But the authors also recognize that planning ahead may not always be feasible and offer a method for making the on-the-spot choices based upon a sound knowledge of the fat content of most common foods.

They provide sample breakfasts, lunches, and dinners that are high in satisfaction and low in fat. They offer coping skills for parties, restaurant eating, supermarket shopping, boredom, loneliness, and other emotional deprivation. The book suggests weighing yourself no more than once a week and doing so in a consistent manner (same amount of clothing, same time of day) so as not to distort your weight loss progress.

Maintenance suggestions are simple and pragmatic: once you reach your ideal body weight, you revise the fat budget, elevating it from 10 percent to 15 percent or 17 percent, using trial and error to arrive at a budget that is both comfortable and maintenance promoting.

A nice inclusion is the suggestion to start children with good eating habits early by easing the entire family into low-fat eating.

NUTRITIONAL EVALUATION   Averaging two days' menus, the caloric level is within the diet's recommendations and low enough to promote gradual weight loss. The nutrients break down as follows:

Carbohydrates	59%
Protein	23%
Fat	18%
Sodium	3,856 milligrams
Fiber	24 grams
Cholesterol	169 milligrams

As the diet's description claims, this is a high-carbohydrate, low-fat diet—fat and cholesterol, in fact, are well below recommended daily maximums. Protein, however, is a little higher than recommended; but because the carbohydrates are high and fat is low, I feel that the protein level is acceptable. Sodium is 38 percent above guidelines; I would suggest cutting the sodium in the book's recipes by at least half.

The diet provides 100 percent of the RDA guidelines for all essential vitamins and minerals except for zinc, which is above two-thirds of the RDA.

PRACTICALITY   This is a user-friendly book, providing a good deal of easily accessible and highly valuable nutritional information, including a table describing the fat content of over 3,000 foods. It presents one of the simplest methods for reducing total fat: counting fat calories. *Choose to Lose* forbids no foods—it just limits those high in fat—making it a realistic program for many people.

ANALYSIS OF 2-DAY MENU FOR FEMALE AGE 35

The Choose To Lose Diet

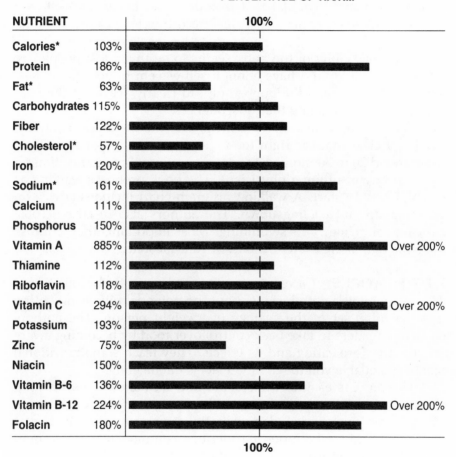

PERCENTAGE OF RA/RM

NUTRIENT		
Calories*	103%	
Protein	186%	
Fat*	63%	
Carbohydrates	115%	
Fiber	122%	
Cholesterol*	57%	
Iron	120%	
Sodium*	161%	
Calcium	111%	
Phosphorus	150%	
Vitamin A	885%	Over 200%
Thiamine	112%	
Riboflavin	118%	
Vitamin C	294%	Over 200%
Potassium	193%	
Zinc	75%	
Niacin	150%	
Vitamin B-6	136%	
Vitamin B-12	224%	Over 200%
Folacin	180%	

100%

*Recommended maximum allowance. Nutrient should not exceed 100%.

LIFESTYLE AND EXERCISE The authors underscore the importance of behavior in achieving healthy eating and weight control. The book asks readers to rethink attitudes toward high-fat foods, to weigh the benefits against the drawbacks. The authors use a number of financial metaphors as illustrations. For example, the way that high-fat food calories rapidly add up is compared to monthly credit card bills. If you don't think about it, the numbers suddenly rise out of control; but if you keep a watchful eye, you can keep those numbers reasonable. The authors also offer a passbook (like those used for savings accounts) that includes food tables, as well as a balance book for keeping a two-week record of total calories and fat calories.

The philosophy of the book seems to be this: Most people are intelligent enough and have enough self-esteem to do what is best for themselves, given the opportunity to clearly see what they are doing and to understand the consequences.

Choose to Lose also discusses the benefits of physical activity, making it clear that the right food choices are not a panacea. They recommend 20 to 30 minutes of aerobic exercise three to five times a week (after consulting a physician). The book proposes walking as the best way to start. A walking program chart includes advice on warming up and cooling down. The authors also discuss aerobic dancing, bicycling, and swimming. Most important, they address the issue of making exercise a part of your lifestyle.

WHY IT WORKS   *Choose to Lose* is based upon fairly solid scientific data, coupled with insight about the potential pitfalls of dieting and the mind-set of the average overweight person. The authors challenge readers to take back control over food by becoming aware of what they are eating and its effects. They teach some nutritional realities to enable you to read food labels intelligently.

The book is easy to understand and facilitates quick learning about the low-fat way of eating. It illustrates a typical day's eating (three meals plus snacks), demonstrating ways to manipulate the fat percentage and total calories in order to accommodate various situations without compromising weight control.

The authors work to break some of the bad habits many dieters become accustomed to, such as skipping meals, starving, and going on binges. This is a positive and encouraging book, teaching not just weight control but general principles about how to become—and stay—healthy through the right food choices.

POTENTIAL DRAWBACKS   This is a diet for people who are highly motivated and willing to be aggressive in their weight management. Being a dietary fat detective—researching the fat content in everything you eat, including restaurant dishes—is no small task. Although this requirement may ensure success for some, its demands on time and energy may present difficulties for others.

A discussion about target heart rate would provide useful information regarding the importance of exercising within one's target heart range. The necessity of fluid replacement during and after exercise is not addressed.

SECOND OPINION   "While the concept of reducing total fat in the diet for weight loss is not new, the Goors' approach of counting fat calories simplifies the process."

—Environmental Nutrition Newsletter

THE EXECUTIVE SUCCESS DIET

by June Roth, M.S.,
and Harvy Ross, M.D.
McGraw Hill Book Company
New York: 1986

ABOUT THE AUTHORS   June Roth, M.S., has a degree in clinical nutrition. She writes a syndicated newspaper column, "Special Diets/Nutrition Hotline," and is the author of more than 30 books on food and nutrition. Harvy Ross, M.D., is a Los Angeles–based psychiatrist and author of *Fighting Depression*. He is a former president of the International College of Applied Nutrition.

WHOM IT'S FOR   As the title suggests, this book offers weight loss and maintenance advice for executives, although the principles may be applied to all working persons or anyone else who needs to be able to perform at a consistently high level of energy and alertness.

OVERVIEW   The diet packages proven nutritional data into a formula to help the reader achieve "health control," as the title of the first chapter suggests. The eight initial tools are:

1. Increasing complex carbohydrates

2. Reducing dietary fats

3. Ensuring sufficient protein

4. Detecting and avoiding excess sodium

5. Learning a "speed method" of calorie counting

6. Learning when to use nutritional supplements

7. Controlling your physical profile (a fast education in medical tests and what they mean)

8. Learning emotional stress reduction techniques

With this foundation, the authors present a diet plan specialized for busy working people, including a five-day work week menu of balanced eating that features a variety of foods to ensure adequate nutrition. The diet can range from 1,000 to 1,500 calories per day, and can be adjusted upward for dieters engaged in more than moderate exercise under their doctor's supervision. The diet also allows for snacks, making such recommendations as an apple break rather than a coffee-and-donut break.

The nutritional recommendations, such as avoiding refined sugar and fat and restricting coffee and alcohol, are backed up with scientific data so that the dieter understands the logic behind the advice. The authors discuss digestion, absorption, and storage of nutrients to help the dieter make sound food choices.

The diet offers specific advice for travel as well as nutritional strategies for such things as a low-fat, low-cholesterol breakfast meeting and a lean "power lunch."

The Executive Success Diet also stresses exercise, and cleverly uses business management principles as a model for setting up exercise, as well as diet and stress management, as priorities.

The book also includes useful related health information, such as a discussion of over-the-counter medicines and other drugs and their effects on nutrition absorption and general health. A review of the Heimlich maneuver is included since, according to the authors, one of the hazards of doing business over a meal is that talking while eating greatly increases the risk of choking.

NUTRITIONAL EVALUATION   Daily calories average out to within the recommendations of the diet. The nutrients break down as follows:

Carbohydrates	55%
Protein	31%
Fat	14%
Sodium	1,510 milligrams
Fiber	21 grams
Cholesterol	262 milligrams

Protein levels are high, but cholesterol is within the recommended goals. On the plus side, carbohydrates are within the recommended levels and fat is less than half of the allowable

ANALYSIS OF 2-DAY MENU FOR FEMALE, AGE 35

The Executive Success Diet

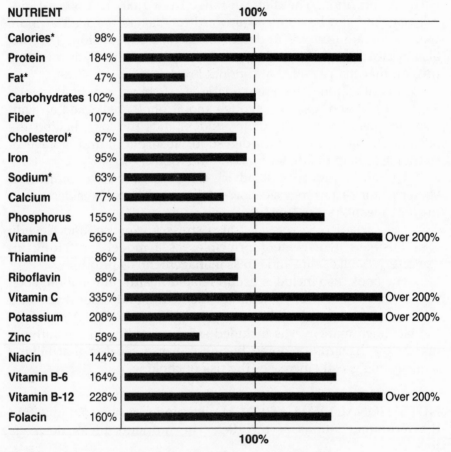

PERCENTAGE OF RA/RM

NUTRIENT		
Calories*	98%	
Protein	184%	
Fat*	47%	
Carbohydrates	102%	
Fiber	107%	
Cholesterol*	87%	
Iron	95%	
Sodium*	63%	
Calcium	77%	
Phosphorus	155%	
Vitamin A	565%	Over 200%
Thiamine	86%	
Riboflavin	88%	
Vitamin C	335%	Over 200%
Potassium	208%	Over 200%
Zinc	58%	
Niacin	144%	
Vitamin B-6	164%	
Vitamin B-12	228%	Over 200%
Folacin	160%	

100%

*Recommended maximum allowance. Nutrient should not exceed 100%.

maximum. Fiber meets the recommended goals and sodium is well below the allowable limit.

Though low in calories, this diet meets 100 percent of the RDA guidelines for all essential micronutrients except for iron, calcium, thiamine, and riboflavin, all of which exceed two-thirds of the RDA, and zinc, which does not. Good food sources of zinc include shellfish and all animal products.

PRACTICALITY   Practicality is part of the theme of *The Executive Success Diet*: How can people with busy and demanding lives control their weight and maintain good health? Thus, the framework of the book allows for the particular demands of the individual. It offers easily accessible information about how to make the right food choices in a wide variety of typical business situations, including hotel stays. Additionally, it provides recipes for simple and wholesome meals at home that even an exhausted executive—or exhausted spouse—can prepare.

LIFESTYLE AND EXERCISE   The lifestyle aspects of this program focus on stress management, describing various methods for dealing with stress without sabotaging diet. The authors emphasize nutritional realities, appealing to the reader's intelligence and common sense so that he or she will have the power to make the right food choices no matter what the situation.

The exercise suggestions have a similar theme: exercise because it's healthful, socially beneficial (doesn't everyone on the board of directors play tennis?), and because it makes you feel good! The book emphasizes the importance of some daily exercise (even if only for 15 minutes), details the most common ways to exercise, and charts the average number of calories burned for each activity.

The authors recommend a doctor's approval and realistic exercise goals with gradual increases to prevent injury or overexertion. They also present the concept of Double-Density Exercise, blocking time for exercise by combining it with other important activities (for example, riding a stationary bike while catching up on business periodicals, taking a walk with a spouse for some quality communication, or exercising with business associates to strengthen a professional relationship). Finally, the book addresses the problem of exercising while on a business trip, suggesting ways to ensure access to a gym or other exercise facility while on the road. It includes an appendix of exercise facilities throughout the United States available to travelers.

WHY IT WORKS   The Executive Success Diet is just that: a program that encourages success-oriented people to use their capacity for self-motivation in order to change their lifestyle to a more health-promoting one. The basic nutritional information accurately reflects current scientific data, and the calorie-range information is both convenient and correct with a simplified method of calorie counting. The book is an easy and fast read—another important factor for people in the fast lane.

POTENTIAL DRAWBACKS   The dietary suggestion of 1000 calories is low and will probably require vitamin and mineral supplements to ensure complete nutrition. These low caloric levels may be unrealistic for any tall or large-frame man. Furthermore, the authors do not provide nutritional information with the recommended recipes, leaving the reader to do some guesswork.

Some of the nutritional information, such as to avoid fatty fish because it is high in saturated fat, is not true. Just the opposite is correct—fish is low in saturated fat, which makes it a healthy food choice. Other important information, such as the advantages of monounsaturated fat and polyunsaturated, is absent. Still other information is somewhat dubious. For example, the authors recommend the use of cheddar cheese (a high-fat food) on a low-fat diet.

The exercise program does not distinguish between people already somewhat active and those for whom exercising will be a radical lifestyle change.

Finally, the aspects of stress management and the psychology of dieting are less detailed than one might expect when one of the authors is a psychiatrist.

SECOND OPINION   "This book could be used as a motivational source for the traveling executive, but should be used in conjunction with professional dietary counseling."

—Current Diet Review

THE FEEL FULL DIET
by Steven R. Peikin, M.D.
Atheneum
New York: 1987

ABOUT THE AUTHOR   Dr. Peikin is an associate professor of medicine and pharmacology at the Jefferson Nutrition Program of the Jefferson Medical College in Philadelphia. He is known for his research on gastrointestinal hormones and the control of food intake.

WHOM IT'S FOR   The author makes the following claim: "If you are overweight, the reasons are most likely physical, *not* psychological." If you overeat you are not responding to your body's hunger-inhibiting mechanism. This program, then, is aimed at those overweight people for whom that is true.

OVERVIEW   The Feel Full Diet is based upon Peikin's research into the connection between hormones and physical hunger. He points out that his research has been published in scientific journals and is supported by a large body of scientific evidence. His focus is on what he refers to as the hunger hormone, cholecystokinin (CCK). According to Peikin, this hormone enters the bloodstream after food is consumed. CCK stimulates the gallbladder and pancreas to deposit bile and secrete digestive enzymes into the intestines, and it also signals the brain when the person has consumed enough food so that the brain can convey the feeling of fullness and the person will stop eating. If this hormonal system is not functioning properly, it is not surprising that the person will eat too much and have difficulty with weight control.

Peikin's diet program, which has been tested in a hospital setting, begins with a discussion of digestion and how it relates to the feeling of fullness or satiety. Then he describes the hormonal inadequacy he believes causes many people to be overweight: they lack adequate cholecystokinin receptors in the intestines so that they do not secrete adequate CCK and thus remain hungry long after they have eaten a sufficient amount of food.

Peikin presents a series of case histories together with a quiz to help dispel commonly held myths about the causes of obesity. He analyzes each myth with the objective of encouraging a positive, guilt-free frame of mind. He then presents his dietary answer to hormonally induced obesity: Eat meals high in complex carbohydrates 20 to 30 minutes *after* eating what Peikin refers to as a Satietizer, a high-protein, high-fat appetizer of no more than a few hundred calories. Examples include Peanut Butter-Honey Balls, Brie with Almonds, Cheesy Crab Dip and Mushroom-Walnut Spread.

This Satietizer, according to Peikin, triggers the CCK receptors, even in people whose receptors are not adequate. These receptors release the CCK hormone, which in turn communicates with the brain, enabling the individual to feel full and satisfied with the low-calorie, high-carbohydrate meal.

Timing is very important with this diet. Once you eat the Satietizer hors d'oeuvre, you must begin the meal within 20 to 30 minutes. Dieters are also encouraged to make mealtime last from 40 to 50 minutes in order to maximize the hormonal effects on the brain and achieve the feeling of fullness. Peikin believes that most Americans eat much too quickly and that this contributes heavily to their present state of poor fitness.

Peikin provides suggestions for a variety of Satietizers, some of which can be employed in emergency situations (such as a sudden lunch invitation). He recommends three meals per day and assures readers that his program will leave the dieter feeling full and satisfied without snacking. In all, he presents two weeks of menus at a caloric level of 1,200 for women and 1,300 for men, along with variations at higher and lower caloric levels. He encourages a multiple one-a-day vitamin and mineral supplement to ensure complete nutrition for anyone striving for weight management.

His program is designed to educate the reader about lifelong healthful eating with dietary fat-cutting tips, dessert-eating tips, and low-fat recipes. He stresses the importance of a commitment to Satietizers and to periodic monitoring of food intake to ensure a successful maintenance of weight loss.

NUTRITIONAL EVALUATION In a two day average, the calories are within an acceptable range, slightly above what the author recommends. Those calories break down as follows:

Carbohydrates 49%
Protein 30%
Fat 21%
Sodium .... 2,368 milligrams
Fiber .... 14 grams
Cholesterol .... 310 milligrams

ANALYSIS OF 2-DAY MENU FOR FEMALE, AGE 35

The Feel Full Diet

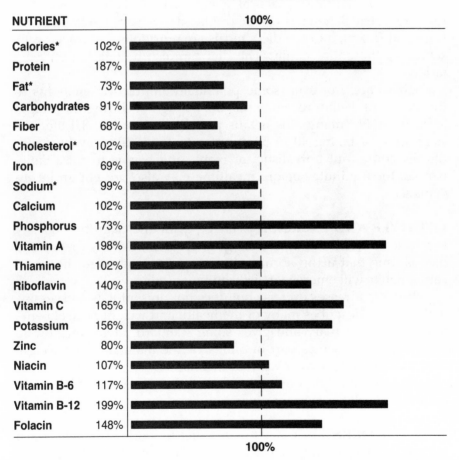

PERCENTAGE OF RA/RM

NUTRIENT		100%
Calories*	102%	
Protein	187%	
Fat*	73%	
Carbohydrates	91%	
Fiber	68%	
Cholesterol*	102%	
Iron	69%	
Sodium*	99%	
Calcium	102%	
Phosphorus	173%	
Vitamin A	198%	
Thiamine	102%	
Riboflavin	140%	
Vitamin C	165%	
Potassium	156%	
Zinc	80%	
Niacin	107%	
Vitamin B-6	117%	
Vitamin B-12	199%	
Folacin	148%	

100%

*Recommended maximum allowance. Nutrient should not exceed 100%.

The protein percentage is too high, even by the pre-1989 RDA—in part because the Satietizers are high in protein. Fat and sodium fall within health goals. Carbohydrates and fiber are low, perhaps a reflection of the author's view that higher carbohydrates and fiber are not the key to weight control. Cholesterol is 3 percent above the recommended daily maximum, but this may not be typical of all days on the diet's meal plans; thus, the cholesterol level could balance out to be below 300 milligrams per day.

All essential micronutrients meet or exceed 100 percent of the RDA except for iron and zinc, which are both above two-thirds.

PRACTICALITY Calorically speaking, this is a flexible program and its aim is extremely practical: a dieter who feels full is less likely to overeat. The Satietizers can be prepared in advance in large quantities and frozen, and the diet's meals are nutritious and thus can be served to the entire family. The diet can also be tailored to vegetarians.

There are, however, some potentially impractical elements to this program. Peikin recommends not eating out during the weight loss phase. For many, this means putting limits on social life. His suggestion of taking 40 to 50 minutes to eat meals may be scientifically sound but unrealistic for many, and having to eat a Satietizer 20 to 30 minutes before mealtime may also present an inconvenience.

LIFESTYLE AND EXERCISE Having made the claim that obesity is a biological and not a psychological problem, Peikin's theory and diet assume that if the hormonal inadequacy is adjusted, healthful eating habits will emerge virtually automatically.

Peikin addresses exercise but does not present it as a necessity. Although he describes many of the health and weight control benefits of aerobic activity and gives some standard advice on how to incorporate exercise as part of a lifestyle, he maintains that weight control is possible with or without exercise.

Behavior modification tips are offered through case history examples and self-assessment quizzes.

WHY IT WORKS In order for this diet to work, the dieter must believe wholeheartedly that it will, that hormonal adjustments can profoundly alter hunger responses and lead to moderate, controlled eating. Given that belief, this program provides a structured framework for losing weight. Fear of hunger can be crippling for overweight people trying to diet. Just the thought of feeling hungry is enough to discourage them. Piekin promises readers that they can feel full without overeating. Trusting that promise alone can have profound results. Peikin backs up the promise with clinical human studies.*

SOME POTENTIAL DRAWBACKS Peikin's assertion that overeating is a biochemical and not a psychological problem may be a gross oversimplification and generalization. Most dietitians who have worked with the obese have often heard the statement, "Sometimes I eat when I'm not even hungry." Surely there are a great many who overeat for comfort and the suppression of emotional difficulties.

While the author encourages exercise, he merely leaves it as an option. Even Peikin himself describes exercise as essential to elevating the body's metabolic rate to ensure weight loss. Without exercise, then, one could reduce calories as per this diet and remain overweight because of an unsatisfactory ratio between fat and lean muscle tissue.

Finally, this book has been criticized for claiming to present original concepts that are not really original. Such criticism, however, does not undermine the effectiveness of the diet.

SECOND OPINION "While this book presents a generally safe and interesting diet plan, it really doesn't say anything new."
—*Current Diet Review*

---

*I tried this approach myself, eating a small high-fat pre-meal, and did subsequently feel less inclined to finish my dinner.

THE I-DON'T-EAT (BUT I CAN'T LOSE) WEIGHT-LOSS PROGRAM

by Steven Jonas, M.D., M.P.H., and
Virginia Aronson, R.D., M.S.
Macmillan Publishing Company
New York: 1989

ABOUT THE AUTHORS   Steven A. Jonas is a professor of community/preventive medicine at the State University of New York at Stony Brook. This diet is based on Dr. Jonas's own personal dietary and exercise transformation. Virginia Aronson is author of nine nutrition books.

WHOM IT'S FOR   This program is for people who don't eat very much yet are inexplicably overweight; Jonas refers to them as the diet-induced overweight. The program is not for children, for pregnant women, or for anyone with a medical problem.

OVERVIEW   "Diets don't work," say the authors. "They are unhealthy, depressing, and ultimately self-defeating." With that in mind, Jonas and Aronson present a weight control program that they suggest is not a weight loss diet in the traditional sense.

They begin by explaining why low-calorie diets don't work for many people. They discuss the issue of fat, differentiating between being overweight and overfat and examining the evolutionary, psychological, and philosophical implications of body fat. "Fat is not," they stress, "a sin." Rather than using weight as a measurement, the book suggests employing the waist-to-hip ratio with a body mass index chart and body measurements. They pay special attention to upper-body fat, often associated with increased risk of heart disease and diabetes. The goals of this diet are not to lose weight and keep it off but to lose fat and then maintain a healthy body-fat percentage.

The program begins with self-evaluation, a series of questions that reveal the dieter's attitudes about issues related to fat. The reader scores and analyzes the answers. Then the authors offer encouragement and ask the reader to examine his or her body image.

The authors return to the self-evaluation process in order to ensure that dieters set reasonable and attainable goals. They suggest that eating habits can be unlearned and new ones gradually learned to take their place.

The authors recommend a low-fat, high-carbohydrate eating plan of moderation, in three distinct phases:

1. A gradual reduction in dietary fat lasting at least four weeks.

2. A steadily reduced fat intake that will achieve desired weight loss over a safe period of time.

3. More food, less fat as a plan for lifelong maintenance.

Although the three phases can be followed in succession, dieters may begin at phase two or even three, depending on their goals and needs. At each phase, the dieter customizes an eating plan in which carbohydrates are the primary food, and meats and other protein sources are complementary food sources. The book offers "fat slashing" tips to ensure ideal meal choices.

The eating plan recommends 55 to 60 percent of calories from carbohydrates; 10 to 15 percent from protein; and no more than 30 percent from fat. Food tables in the book illustrate exactly what that means in terms of meal choices and their effects on a day's menu. The authors add information about nutrition, dietary variety, cholesterol, and refined sugars, then share ways to make good food selections in a variety of potentially difficult eating situations.

They emphasize daily exercise as a key part of any weight loss plan and provide tips not only for changing eating behavior but also for conquering the emotional aspects of losing and controlling weight. The book devotes special attention to the dietary considerations of women, including vitamin and mineral deficiencies, hidden dietary caffeine and its ability to aggravate premenstrual syndrome in some women, and the specific nutritional needs of pregnant women and women over 50.

The authors devote a good deal of attention to giving the reader an ongoing pep talk, encouraging the reader to take responsibility and then to take action.

NUTRITIONAL EVALUATION   This diet does not present specific daily menus, meal plans, or recipes. Thus, it would be impossible to give a breakdown of micro- or macronutrients, since every dieter will make different choices within the guidelines. The diet does, however, provide food lists representing the four basic food groups: (1) fruits and vegetables, (2) bread and cereal, (3) milk and cheese, (4) meat and meat alternatives.

In groups 1, 2, and 4 this diet's recommendations are completely within a safe and healthful range. In the milk and cheese group, the book suggests three to four servings per day. This would be advisable only if those are servings of either nonfat or 1% dairy products.

PRACTICALITY   The book is easy to read; the authors make complex issues accessible and the information usable. The voice of moderation, backed by some scientific insights, results in a realistic plan for many overweight individuals. Goals are short-range, and improvement at any speed is one of the primary goals. Tips are clear and useful for everything from fat substitutes to eating out, from seizing inner motivation to nighttime eating. The flexibility of the diet enables the dieter to feel a sense of control, responsibility, and freedom.

On the down side, the authors' dining-out suggestion to bring along a 10-page list of foods' fat content is impractical. Prior knowledge of the fat content of common foods would be a much simpler and more usable approach.

LIFESTYLE AND EXERCISE   The book's self-evaluation questionnaires supply a nice foundation for the behavioral aspects of weight control. The authors ask the reader to evaluate eating habits and associated feelings, and then they provide methods for applying that awareness toward self-improvement. Additionally, the authors deliver a continual flow of encouragement—which most dieters cannot get enough of, especially those for whom dieting has been a series of failures.

Like the diet, the book's Ideal Exercise Plan is divided into three phases. The program centers around pace walking, a combination of leg stride and arm swing at an aerobic pace. The three phases are as follows:

1. Novice pace walking, an introduction to regular aerobic exercise.

2. Regular exercise, developing skill and ability.

3. New You formula at one of three levels, based upon age and maximum heart rate.

The authors present pace walking as an exercise as healthful as jogging or swimming and as the safest and most universally accessible, especially to the overweight. They provide tips on everything from buying the right athletic shoes for pace walking to finding time for exercise and maximizing that time. They also address issues of resistance and explain how to "Get out of your own way and let the athlete within emerge." As with all aspects of this book, self-evaluation is a major component of the exercise program, and the reader is given the freedom to choose what is most comfortable.

WHY IT WORKS   The scientific data upon which this program is based are accurate and consistent with the recommendations and findings of a number of professional health organizations. Low-fat, high-carbohydrate eating of a variety of foods coupled with exercise is the most sensible way to achieve weight control. The program is not only flexible and comprehensive, but it advocates gradual and thus realistic change in diet and other habits.

The authors address with clarity and depth all of the important elements of a weight control program. Especially insightful is their discussion of why fad diets don't work over the long haul even if the dieter follows them to the letter.

SOME POTENTIAL DRAWBACKS   This program is not for the dieter who needs an external structure. While some people may enjoy the freedom and self-control this diet advocates, others may not have the self-motivation to succeed. Although you should never underestimate yourself, you should also be realistic about your limitations.

While the diet plan is sensible, its use of food lists and the necessity of mapping out meals may be a hindrance to some people. A few basic menus would have been helpful for those dieters who prefer to follow a ready-made eating plan.

SECOND OPINIONS   "This book is recommended to the general public as a guide and motivational tool when starting a diet and fitness program."   *—Current Diet Review*

"The I-Don't-Eat (But I Can't Lose) Weight-Loss Program is an easy-to-read, accurate and balanced eating plan for people trying to lose weight or merely trying to begin a more healthful way of eating."

—Environmental Nutrition Newsletter

THE I-QUIT-SMOKING DIET

by Janice Alpert, M.A.
Contemporary Books
Chicago; 1988

ABOUT THE AUTHOR   Alpert is a psychotherapist specializing in eating disorders at Chicago's Guidance and Counseling Center.

WHOM IT'S FOR   This book is designed specifically for people who have quit smoking and want to avoid the potential weight gain that often accompanies the conquering of the nicotine habit. It is also for smokers who want to quit smoking but are afraid of the weight gain. According to the American Lung Association, of all the Americans who kick the habit, one-third lose weight, one-third maintain their current weight, and one-third gain weight. The target audience of *The I-Quit-Smoking Diet* is the last third—and even a segment of the second third, because it encourages weight loss for the already overweight ex-smoker.

OVERVIEW   The book begins with a study of what the author sees as the human potential for change. She encourages readers not to underestimate their own capacity, to listen to the "inner voice or gut instinct," and to recognize the fact that "change requires practice and effort." Then Alpert takes readers through an examination of the effects of smoking and the effects—both alleged and real—of nicotine withdrawal as the body reacts to the cessation of smoking.

She begins with the chemical effects of smoking on the body. These may be familiar to many, but it is nonetheless important to reconsider them as a motivating factor in quitting smoking, especially when underscored by the fact that most of the degeneration associated with smoking is reversible.

Alpert then considers the role of nicotine in speeding up metabolism, along with the possibility that quitting smoking slows down the body's metabolic rate, causing the former smoker to gain weight without changing diet. Alpert asserts that this connection does not explain weight gain, that nicotine's effect on metabolism is not significant. There are other potential reasons, she explains, why former smokers tend to have a particular vulnerability to weight gain. These factors include the emotional/social aspects of cigarette smoking and the effect of nicotine on taste buds: nicotine deadens the taste sensation, suppressing the desire for sweet foods. When taste buds come alive again after the smoker gives up tobacco, it is not surprising that strong cravings for sweet foods may arise.

Another connection between quitting smoking and weight gain explored here is that of habit. Many smokers light up right after a meal. Without the cigarette to punctuate the end of a meal, many former smokers find themselves eating more than they used to. Finally, and perhaps most profoundly, Alpert suggests that eating more after quitting smoking is an attempt to suppress uncomfortable feelings that may have previously been suppressed through smoking.

The book suggests ways to handle these problems without consuming more calories. The first step, according to the author, is to identify the emotional triggers and then devise coping mechanisms and strategies. Alpert recommends the use of a journal and self-reflective writing exercises to discover and diagnose feelings and emotional triggers. She presents the reader with a variety of alternatives to cigarettes and excess food. The information is described in detail and then summarized in the form of a "feelings chart."

Alpert emphasizes the importance of taking action on your insight—implementing the positive alternatives, not just thinking about them. She suggests the creation of a "Put Yourself First Chart" in order to ensure that your needs are always a priority.

This process begins, according to the author, with the recognition and acceptance of the fact that the smoker perceives that to stop smoking is a loss. It can feel like the end of a friendship—a destructive friendship, yes, but its ending can still be emotionally traumatic. Alpert encourages readers to accept that they are going through a period of mourning. She recommends constructive ways to mourn so that ex-smokers can achieve symbolic as well as physical closure to the relationship with cigarettes. This process is followed by a symbolic personal transformation in which the ex-smoker sets goals about the kind of person he or she will strive to be without the dependency on cigarettes.

Having dealt with the psychological and emotional issues of smoking and its cessation, Alpert then presents an eating program for the ex-smoker. She begins with a general discussion of a moderate lifestyle: proper eating coupled with moderate aerobic exercise leads to weight control. She provides practical information about basic nutrition and then describes a food plan based upon the guidelines of the American Cancer Society and reflecting data about the vitamins and minerals most important to smokers and recent ex-smokers. The eating plan stresses three areas:

1. Foods that can ease nicotine withdrawal, based upon the theory that keeping urine alkaline allows nicotine in the bloodstream to leave the body slowly, thus preventing sudden harsh cravings. Foods for this purpose include vegetables, most fruit juices, and milk products. Poultry, eggs, seafood, and other acid-forming foods are limited during this period. Foods rich in vitamins B and C are emphasized.

2. Low caloric levels (1,200 for women, 1,600 for men) tailored to gradual weight loss (one to two pounds per week) or maintenance needs.

3. A goal of good lifetime eating habits with moderation as the cornerstone. The author provides three weeks of sample menus, encouraging the dieter to learn how to eat moderately.

NUTRITIONAL EVALUATION   Analysis of an average of two days' menus showed a caloric level significantly lower than the author's own recommendations. This level is too low, especially for an ex-smoker with increased needs for certain key nutrients. Making portions slightly larger and taking a daily multiple vitamin and mineral supplement (not exceeding 100 percent of the RDA) should remedy this problem. The calories break down as follows:

```
Carbohydrates ........................... 56%
Protein .................................. 24%
Fat ...................................... 20%
Sodium ................................... 1,474 milligrams
Fiber .................................... 13 grams
Cholesterol .............................. 136 milligrams
```

Protein is higher than recommended goals—and considerably above those suggested by the author. Carbohydrates, however, are encouragingly high, and fat and cholesterol are encouragingly low.

ANALYSIS OF 2-DAY MENU FOR FEMALE, AGE 35

The I-Quit-Smoking Diet

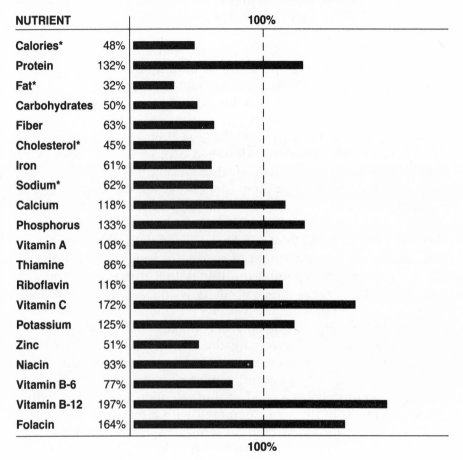

NUTRIENT	PERCENTAGE OF RA/RM
Calories*	48%
Protein	132%
Fat*	32%
Carbohydrates	50%
Fiber	63%
Cholesterol*	45%
Iron	61%
Sodium*	62%
Calcium	118%
Phosphorus	133%
Vitamin A	108%
Thiamine	86%
Riboflavin	116%
Vitamin C	172%
Potassium	125%
Zinc	51%
Niacin	93%
Vitamin B-6	77%
Vitamin B-12	197%
Folacin	164%

100%

*Recommended maximum allowance. Nutrient should not exceed 100%.

Fiber falls substantially short of the recommended minimum intake. Again, an increase in portion size with an emphasis on whole grains should improve that number.

All essential micronutrients meet or exceed 100 percent of the RDA guidelines except for thiamine, niacin, and vitamin B-6, which meet at least two-thirds of the RDA, and iron and zinc, which do not. That the diet does not meet the 100 percent level for all of the B-vitamins is surprising since the author emphasizes their importance to the recovery of the ex-smoker. Increasing portion sizes of whole wheat products should provide the diet higher levels of these important nutrients. Foods rich in iron include lean meats, dried beans and peas, whole grains, and enriched cereals. Zinc is plentiful in all animal products and in shellfish.

PRACTICALITY   This book is easy to read and its advice is reasonable. Weight loss is gradual and all food groups are represented so that dieters can satisfy their individual tastes.

Cigarette smoking, we now know, is among the hardest (if not *the* hardest) addiction to overcome, and many people resign themselves to weight gain as the inevitable side effect of giving up the tobacco habit. But Alpert has designed a program that should be workable for most ex-smokers, so that kicking the habit can be the beginning of a more healthful existence and not the trading of one bad habit for another.

LIFESTYLE AND EXERCISE   Alpert gives thorough coverage to the critical lifestyle component of successful weight control, detailing strategies for overcoming the things that trigger smoking and overeating. Her suggested feelings diary is an excellent tool for identifying and dealing with the variety of emotional issues behind smoking and eating. It not only encourages coping but also promotes independence. Addressing the issue of loss and mourning can be very useful. Awareness is crucial to behavior modification; you cannot correct behavior until you have identified it.

The author devotes a good deal of attention to exercise, with a strong argument in its favor (tempered with a recommendation for medical supervision), and then presents a realistic approach for ex-smokers. This begins with an activity profile questionnaire to help select the best form of exercise. The book's activity plan contains four components:

1. A walking plan

2. Aerobic activities

3. Optional activities (anything from gardening to bowling or square dancing)

4. Relaxation techniques

As this list suggests, Alpert's concern is not limited to the metabolic and calorie-burning effects of aerobic exercise, but to the general state of well-being that an active life can produce. As with eating, the book recommends a balanced, moderate, and realistic approach to exercise and urges the reader to pursue as much self-awareness as possible, to monitor results, and to feel good about them.

WHY IT WORKS   This book goes a long way toward allaying the fears of smokers who are reluctant to quit or ex-smokers who feel they cannot make it without gaining weight. The food program is, for the most part, nutritionally sound and should enable the individual to achieve weight control through good food choices and moderation. Alpert's discussion of macronutrients is clear, concise, and—most important—convincing.

The emphasis on drinking a lot of fluid is a good one, since adequate liquid intake is essential to proper digestion and since hunger and thirst are often confused, leading people to eat when what they really crave is a glass of water.

The book's tone is positive, but the author does not understate the severity either of the smoking habit or of the potential difficulties in quitting without the residual weight gain. In essence, her message is this: You have a tough job ahead of you—and every reason to believe that you can make it. Confidence is perhaps the most meaningful element in these pages.

SOME POTENTIAL DRAWBACKS   Some of the nutritional information is inaccurate. For example, Alpert's discussion of cholesterol states that HDL (good) cholesterol cleans plaque out of the arteries. In fact, HDL carries cholesterol to the liver, a desired result that contributes to healthy arteries but is not an actual artery-cleansing process. The suggestion that antacid tablets are a good source of calcium for the body is a myth. Calcium requires an antacid environment in order to be absorbed properly by the body, and antacids create the opposite environment.

The book also makes some omissions. The author's discussion of dietary fats lacks current data about saturated, polyunsaturated, and monounsaturated oils. The discussion of the importance of fiber neither differentiates water-soluble from water-insoluble fiber nor gives lists of good sources of either type.

The most consequential oversights are the lack of a maintenance program and the lack of any recommendations for eating out or for any other particularly difficult eating situations.

Finally, the theory about alkaline urine helping to regulate the discharge of nicotine and reduce cravings is not supported by adequate scientific data. However, since the foods recommended in connection with the theory are healthful, the risk/benefit ratio is in favor of accepting the theory on faith.

SECOND OPINION "If used as part of a smoking-cessation class, with guidance from a dietitian for better food selections, the book would be helpful at guiding the user through the emotional pitfalls of successful smoking cessation and weight management."

—Current Diet Review

Living Lean by Choosing More

by Cheryl Jennings-Sauer
M.A., R.D., L.D.
Taylor Publishing Company
Dallas, Texas: 1989

ABOUT THE AUTHOR   A registered and licensed dietitian, Jennings-Sauer holds a master's degree in nutrition and teaches at the Austin Community College. She is director of the Living Lean Program, provided to the employees of participating companies such as IBM and medical centers and based upon the principles in this book.

WHOM IT'S FOR   This book is for those the author refers to as "moderately overfat people" who are looking for a safe and workable technique to lose fat with little or no professional monitoring. The program can be useful for the compulsive dieter who wants to break the cycle of losing and gaining and, at the same time, to rebuild physical and psychological health. It may also be a good program for anyone who is already in good health and at an ideal weight and is looking for an effective method of maintenance.

The philosophy of this diet is to achieve goals through small successes. The author offers the formula Q_2FIT, which stands for *quality control, quantity control, fitness, initiative*, and *timing*. The book encourages consultation with a physician before adopting a high-fiber, nutrient-dense, low-fat diet in tandem with aerobic exercise. It is difficult to imagine any M.D. objecting to this plan.

OVERVIEW   Jennings-Sauer has devised an eight-week program that includes behaviorally oriented steps toward modifying diet and lifestyle in order to achieve a weight loss goal. For the first week, the program encourages the dieter to consider cutting down (not *out*) those favorite foods responsible for obesity and suggests some behavioral exercises, including:

- Listing the immediate and long-term effects of improving your health and appearance.

- Visualizing how you will look.

- Writing down potential stumbling blocks along with some creative ways to mitigate them.

- Signing, in front of a witness, a participant agreement confirming your commitment to following the program.

- Practicing positive thought control.

Dieters are encouraged to do a "pantry inventory," during which they read the labels and note the sugar and salt content of foods, and to begin a food diary on a form provided in the book. The first week also includes the advice to start walking (after a doctor's approval).

During the second week, the dieter analyzes the food diary and begins measuring the duration of meals and the time lapse between them, with an objective of spacing meals no more than four hours apart to avoid severe dips in blood sugar. The second week also introduces a Q&A behavioral modification exercise, along with important information about the benefits of dietary fiber and its best sources. *Living Lean* also offers methods for how to handle hunger, including small snacks, careful "grazing" at parties, and lunches that can satisfy you until dinner.

For the balance of the eight weeks, the dieter builds on this foundation:

- *Week three*: The whys and hows of exercise.

- *Week four*: A guide to good foods, those that will enhance health and help control weight; where to get them and how much to eat of them.

- *Week five*: How to increase metabolism and why.

- *Week six*: An individualized eating plan design; determining the maximum calories you can eat and still enable your body to burn fat and maintain lean muscle tissue.

- *Week seven*: Identifying stress and learning ways to reduce it; behavioral strategies, such as written exercises that help you gain objectivity; physical strategies, such as aerobic exercise as a stress reducer; and nutritional strategies, such as avoiding excess refined sugar.

- *Week eight*: Motivation through assessing the positive change you've made during the first seven weeks, along with additional positive changes as attainable goals.

After these initial eight weeks, the program suggests building on your successes—large or modest—and keeping up your progress, always looking for ways to modify, improve, and incorporate positive change into your lifestyle.

NUTRITIONAL EVALUATION   Analysis of a two-day average eating plan came to slightly more calories than are suggested by the author. This may be too high for some people to lose weight, although the fat percentage is sufficiently small to encourage weight loss in most.

Carbohydrates	57%
Protein	24%
Fat	19%
Sodium	2,221 milligrams
Fiber	32 grams
Cholesterol	107 milligrams

Fiber is healthfully high, in part because of the adequate percentage of carbohydrates. Fat and cholesterol are happily low (cholesterol, in fact, is approximately one-third of the allowable level). Protein is a little on the high side, but because carbohydrates are above 55 percent and fat is low, I do not find this objectionable. This diet provides 100 percent of the RDA guidelines for all essential vitamins and minerals.

ANALYSIS OF 2-DAY MENU FOR FEMALE, AGE 35

Living Lean by Choosing More

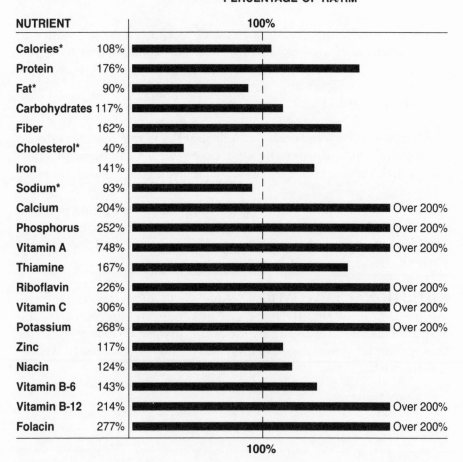

PERCENTAGE OF RA/RM

NUTRIENT		100%
Calories*	108%	
Protein	176%	
Fat*	90%	
Carbohydrates	117%	
Fiber	162%	
Cholesterol*	40%	
Iron	141%	
Sodium*	93%	
Calcium	204%	Over 200%
Phosphorus	252%	Over 200%
Vitamin A	748%	Over 200%
Thiamine	167%	
Riboflavin	226%	Over 200%
Vitamin C	306%	Over 200%
Potassium	268%	Over 200%
Zinc	117%	
Niacin	124%	
Vitamin B-6	143%	
Vitamin B-12	214%	Over 200%
Folacin	277%	Over 200%

100%

*Recommended maximum allowance. Nutrient should not exceed 100%.

PRACTICALITY   The tips and suggestions in this book are useful, simple, and, for many people, easy to implement. For example, the author provides easy ways to turn low-fiber meals into high-fiber meals. She also encourages readers to set their own pace for success and, where applicable, to build on what already may work for them in some aspect of weight control.

Refreshingly, Jennings-Sauer omits negative words like *diet*, *cheat*, and the dreaded *will power*. The program allows for flexibility in terms of individual tastes, diversity in nutritional needs, and ways of adapting to various lifestyles. Finally, the book goes beyond practicing weight control just for the sake of looking good. The author seems more concerned with the health and well-being of her readers, recommending, for example, that they quit smoking—an action that can make eating modifications more difficult in the short term but general health much better in the long run.

The only potential impracticality of this program is the record keeping, which may be a time-consuming turn-off for some people. (It is conceivable that you could utilize this diet *without* the record keeping.)

LIFESTYLE AND EXERCISE   Behavioral modification is the cornerstone of this program. The lessons provide good opportunities to identify the reasons why eating right is difficult and then to devise ways to overcome the problem. Although thoughtfully structured, they allow for the uniqueness of each person.

The author emphasizes the importance of exercise in any approach to weight control and good health, providing guidelines on safety, medical supervision, and frequency. She states, for example, that while exercising three times per week will promote cardiovascular improvement, muscle tone, calorie burning, and the mental lift of endorphins, research has found that exercising four or five times per week burns significantly more fat. Thus, for fat burning, frequency of exercise is more important than duration. Jennings-Sauer also discusses the biochemistry of fat burning, offering some important information about nutritional deficiencies that can undermine fat burning and ways to avoid them. Finally, and perhaps most important, the author supplies words of inspiration to help in the pursuit of the most crucial element of any consistent exercise regimen: self-motivation.

WHY IT WORKS   The book is readable and accessible. Its humor gives it an upbeat feel. Each chapter begins with a list of its subjects, enabling the reader to zero in on any points of special interest.

The program is pragmatic, offering a combination of inspiration and information to make what for many may seem a Mission Impossible—weight control—seem attainable. It is a program that stresses the importance of a balanced approach to weight control and health: nutrition, exercise, stress management, and behavioral modification.

The high-carbohydrate, low-fat food recommendations are a safe, practical, and effective way to lose weight and keep it off. The recipes are good, the explanations are clear, and the discussions of exercise and stress management are particularly thorough. The goals are not centered around weight loss but on the actions that will bring about that result. The author advises avoiding the scale, a good idea since most people tend to overdo weighing themselves and consequently become discouraged before they give themselves an opportunity to succeed. Dwelling on daily weight changes can only get in the way of taking the actions that lead to weight loss.

POTENTIAL DRAWBACKS   The program asks dieters to do a lot of record keeping, and though the intent is self-reflective and the practice can be eye-opening, this requirement may be an inconvenience to some people.

Also, although I applaud her advice to quit smoking and her omission of caffeine from menus, cutting out caffeine and nicotine while modifying one's diet all in an eight-week period may be a bit too ambitious for some people.

SECOND OPINIONS   "Well, someone finally got it right! Now if we can only *de-program* American dieters and get them to embody Cheryl Jennings-Sauer's message!"

—Current Diet Review

"*Living Lean* is a one-stop shopper for anyone who wants to lose weight *and* get healthier."

—American Health Magazine

THE NEW AMERICAN DIET

by Sonja L. Connor, M.S., R.D.,
and William E. Connor, M.D.
Simon & Schuster
New York: 1986

ABOUT THE AUTHORS   Sonja Connor is a research assistant and professor of clinical nutrition at Oregon Health Science University in Portland. Dr. William Connor is chief of endocrinology, metabolism, and clinical nutrition at the Oregon Health Sciences University. He is a member of the Food and Nutrition Board of the National Academy of Sciences and has worked in the heart disease prevention field for over 20 years. Both authors were personally involved in a five-year research study of 233 American families (funded by the National Heart, Lung, and Blood Institute) that examined the effects of diet on weight and illness. This book is based upon that research.

WHOM IT'S FOR   This program can work for anyone interested in weight control and/or general good health. You need not be overweight to benefit from the nutritional advice in this book.

OVERVIEW   The authors begin with a discussion of the most perilous problems related to the typical American diet and its effect on health and well-being. They survey the various diseases that can result from both over- and underconsumption of food and then present the potential benefits of positive nutritional change. Their approach is a three-step progression, to be accomplished at the dieter's own pace, that gradually shifts eating habits from high-fat, high-cholesterol, high-salt, and low-carbohydrate foods to the precise opposite.

Phase One focuses on substitution, demonstrating simple ways to replace high-fat, salty foods with low-fat, low-sodium alternatives. The authors also explain how to substitute lean meats, fish, and poultry for their fatty counterparts. A key feature is a Cholesterol Saturated-Fat Index (CSI), a set of easily readable charts that help the reader begin to perceive foods according to their health values.

Phase Two introduces new recipes, including healthful approaches to ethnic cooking, featuring Mexican, Oriental, and Middle Eastern/Mediterranean flavors. At this point, the authors suggest a more radical reduction in high-fat meats and fatty cheese products. They discuss the traditional sandwich and point out ways to make major modifications in content while maintaining culinary quality.

The authors assure the reader that following the prescriptions of Phase Two represents a major step, and that even if you were to stop there, this in itself would be a significant accomplishment. However, they urge you *not* to stop there.

Phase Three is an entirely new way of eating. The goal of the diet: "defensive eating for disease prevention." At this point, meat is deemphasized, while complex carbohydrates become the staple.

The authors prefer the body mass index, rather than weight charts, to determine ideal body weight goals, although they do provide the Metropolitan Life weight charts for those who feel more comfortable consulting them. They advise caloric restrictions of 1,000 calories for women and 2,000 for men in order to achieve a loss of one to two pounds per week. These caloric limitations are to apply only until the dieter loses enough weight to "feel good" about himself or herself. Then it's back to the core program starting at Phase Two without caloric restrictions; this can minimize any subsequent weight gain.

The book furnishes tips and information about how to maintain healthy eating habits during special occasions. The authors present scenarios along with practical and nonconfrontational remedies.

The New American Diet gives special advice for pregnant women and breast-feeding mothers and basic guidelines for infant feeding. It also provides modifications to accommodate vegetarians.

NUTRITIONAL EVALUATION The gradual dietary alterations focus primarily on the reduction of fat and cholesterol and the increase of complex carbohydrates. The nutritional model of the New American Diet thus looks like this:

PHASE	CHOLESTEROL	FAT	COMPLEX CARBOHYDRATES
One	300–350 milligrams	35%	50%
Two	200 milligrams	25%	60%
Three	100 milligrams	20%	65%

The reduction of fat to 20 percent of total daily calories represents about half of the fat consumption of the average American. In addition, the *saturated* fat consumption is reduced to less than 6 percent, sodium is down (2,000 milligrams per day) and fiber is up to 45–60 grams.

The average of a two-day menu from Phase Two of this diet found the calories within a reasonable range (the book itself makes no caloric restrictions). Those calories break down as follows:

```
Carbohydrates ............................ 63%
Protein .................................. 14%
Fat ...................................... 23%
Sodium ................................... 2,259 milligrams
Fiber .................................... 24 grams
Cholesterol .............................. 74 milligrams
```

All of these numbers are within recommended goals. These percentages reflect an ideal eating program that more people should strive to achieve. Additionally, all essential vitamins and minerals meet or exceed 100 percent of the RDA except for vitamin A, calcium, and zinc, all of which exceed two-thirds of the RDA.

PRACTICALITY   With five years of research behind this diet, it is not surprising that the recommendations are offered in a realistic and accessible fashion. The gradual, self-paced style of the program can alleviate much of the pressure dieters often feel and also help promote the essential idea that these nutritional changes are not stopgap measures but the beginning of a permanent lifestyle shift.

The dieter has choices—a very important component of any long-term plan. You can, for example, choose to increase the intake of red meat beyond the recommended level, but only by trading off some other high-fat, high-cholesterol food, such as a chocolate dessert.

The recipes provided in the book are relatively easy to prepare and can help mitigate feelings of deprivation. The authors also include advice for a variety of situations, giving the diet a great deal of flexibility.

On the downside, the first two phases of the diet may require an increase in home cooking for some, which may be a minor inconvenience in the pursuit of long-term weight control and good health.

ANALYSIS OF 2-DAY MENU FOR FEMALE, AGE 35

The New American Diet

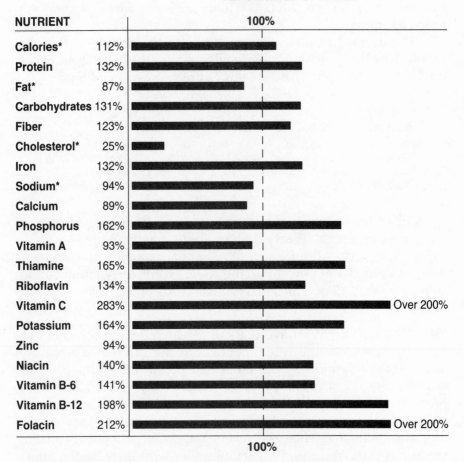

NUTRIENT		PERCENTAGE OF RA/RM
Calories*	112%	
Protein	132%	
Fat*	87%	
Carbohydrates	131%	
Fiber	123%	
Cholesterol*	25%	
Iron	132%	
Sodium*	94%	
Calcium	89%	
Phosphorus	162%	
Vitamin A	93%	
Thiamine	165%	
Riboflavin	134%	
Vitamin C	283%	Over 200%
Potassium	164%	
Zinc	94%	
Niacin	140%	
Vitamin B-6	141%	
Vitamin B-12	198%	
Folacin	212%	Over 200%

100%

*Recommended maximum allowance. Nutrient should not exceed 100%.

LIFESTYLE AND EXERCISE The book contains a number of quizzes that can help readers compare their own eating habits with more ideal habits. Such awareness may not at first seem crucial, but many overweight people lack an accurate perspective on what their present eating habits really are and in what ways they need to be modified. These quizzes can also help dieters gauge their progress and reinforce confidence.

The New American Diet takes complex nutritional data and makes them user friendly. The Cholesterol-Saturated Fat Index gives the reader a single figure by which to rate foods in terms of their effect on blood cholesterol, atherosclerosis, and body weight. Food lists inform the reader of the realities of hidden fats and are accompanied with methods of identifying hidden fat and decreasing it in the diet.

The program engages the dieter's commitment through the use of weekly and monthly goal-oriented contracts, then guides and educates the dieter through more than 300 low-fat recipes. This diet uses food preparation as a major cornerstone of behavior modification. The philosophy is this: You cannot hide the fat if you do the cooking yourself. You have to face fats.

The New American Diet lists the lifestyle, weight control, and other health benefits of aerobic exercise. The authors do not, however, believe it necessary to check your heart rate or to exercise yourself "out of breath." As with diet, the authors suggest modest beginnings and gradual change toward a realistic goal of exercise.

WHY IT WORKS   The book is clearly written and the major points and goals are well presented. The information is sound, accurate, and based on well-researched data. The diet is comprehensive. Weight control is one part of a much larger and more important goal of overall good health. Since this is a long-term—lifelong—goal, the dieter is less vulnerable to the frustration and surrender often associated with losing weight for the single goal of looking more attractive.

The deemphasis of meat in favor of complex carbohydrates can help prevent the hunger that often accompanies a diet. Fruits, vegetables, grains, and legumes tend to be more filling and engage the chewing mechanism more than all but the toughest meats. All advice is backed up by scientific fact.

The diet allows for flexibility—and, on a limited basis, sweets—to reduce the potential feelings of deprivation. Weight loss occurs gradually, as a direct result of behavioral changes, so the dieter gains independence and does not come to rely on an outwardly imposed structure.

POTENTIAL DRAWBACKS   The latitude allowed in the program, while a generally good idea, may mean that some dieters will take a long time to achieve their weight loss goals, using trial and error at various caloric levels.

Also, the authors recommend exercise but present it as an option and not a necessity. Although arm twisting rarely helps the overweight individual, the authors may be misleading readers by suggesting that a change in diet without an increase in physical activity can ensure weight control and improved overall health.

There are other somewhat erroneous points in the book. For example, the authors describe monounsaturated fats as nutritionally neutral—a contradiction of recent data suggesting that monounsaturated fats in moderate amounts can *lower* LDL cholesterol.

There are also some inconsistencies. At one point the authors suggest 800 to 1,200 calories as an acceptable range for weight loss. Later, however, they argue (correctly) against any diets under 1,000 calories.

These inaccuracies and inconsistencies are, however, relatively minor and do not diminish the program's effectiveness.

SECOND OPINION   "Finally, a diet that is not for masochists alone! The authors of this book understand that sheer willpower and determination only last for a short time, and that in order for a diet to be successful it must be reasonable. The New American Diet is just that. . . . This book belongs on every family's shelf. It is a great reference book, cookbook, and meal planner."

—*Current Diet Review*

NOT ANOTHER DIET BOOK: A RIGHT-BRAIN PROGRAM FOR SUCCESSFUL WEIGHT MANAGEMENT

Bobbe Sommer, Ph.D.
Hunter House
Claremont, California: 1987

ABOUT THE AUTHOR   Bobbe Sommer is a licensed marriage and family counselor and a motivational speaker.

WHOM IT'S FOR   This book is for those willing to recognize the role that the mind plays in the process of weight management. Dr. Sommer believes that nutritional advice, no matter how scientifically valid, fails to address the central issue of obesity, which is psychological. This book presents a psychological approach to weight control.

OVERVIEW   *Not Another Diet Book* begins by arguing that food choices are not the dominant reason why people are overweight, that only through psychological changes can an overweight individual lose weight and keep it off.

Sommer invokes the theory of the right versus the left brain. The right brain, she contends, is the intuitive, holistic, visionary half; the left hemisphere is intellectual, verbal, abstract, and analytical. She also distinguishes between the unconscious, subconscious, and conscious aspects of the brain, asserting that by getting in touch with the subconscious, you can learn to reprogram the powerful subconscious thoughts that so often control behavior. Sommer calls her approach the OMS Method: Obtain, Maintain, and Sustain your desired weight.

The program devotes little attention to an actual diet or exercise program, recommending instead that such measures be under the supervision of a doctor. Sommer offers a standard method for determining ideal body weight. The book emphasizes using internal resources to overcome the destructive eating habits responsible for a weight problem and asserts that lifestyle changes from *within* are the best way for anyone to overcome overweight. Using case histories to illustrate many of her points, Dr. Sommer points out some of the kinds of destructive thinking that result in eating and weight problems. For example, she suggests that many women fear losing weight because they anticipate that others will then raise their expectations of them. Men, she says, fear that losing weight means losing power. "He really throws his weight around" is a common expression that supports this idea.

Sommer's six-week program, designed to help people overcome the psychological barriers to weight control, comprises what she calls Reflective Relearning (RR). This, according to Sommer, is a method of "staying in your right brain" through meditative exercises. Its purpose is to help you get in touch with that part of your mind so that you can eventually reprogram it.

Reflective Relearning begins with deep breathing and relaxation, then adds a self-chosen mantra (a word or sentence to repeat while relaxing). This relaxation enables you to dig deep into your past, eventually recalling memories as far back as birth. The idea is to get to the psychological root of your eating disorder and make the necessary adjustments. The most difficult aspect of this technique, according to Sommer, is placating the left hemisphere of the brain, which will often complain that this process is boring, worthless nonsense.

Where Sommer does discuss issues of food choices, she dispels some popular myths (for example, that margarine contains fewer calories than butter) and advocates a natural, high-fiber, low-fat diet. She recommends a number of the enrollment and organized diet programs evaluated in this book.

NUTRITIONAL EVALUATION   This book makes no specific dietary recommendations.

PRACTICALITY   According to Sommer, Reflective Relearning need take only 10 minutes per day. This suggests the utmost in practicality.

LIFESTYLE AND EXERCISE   Behavioral modification is the foundation of this program. Its aim is to help the individual change behavior in order to successfully lose weight and keep it off, no matter what challenges may be encountered. *Not Another Diet Book* stresses adapting to unpleasant situations in a constructive, rather than self-destructive, manner and goes into detail on such issues as the difference between hunger and appetite—appetite is linked strongly to emotions, while hunger is a true physical sensation.

Sommer recommends exercise under the supervision of a doctor. She gives a number of sound reasons for exercising and provides some tips for the overweight exerciser, such as finding an exercise class where at least some of the other people are also overweight in order to avoid comparisons that lead to discouragement. Her other exercise recommendations are pragmatic, based upon the generally accepted view of the nutritional and medical communities: exercise must be aerobic, last 20 to 30 minutes per session, and create a heart rate within 60 to 80 percent of your target heart rate. She emphasizes safety and practicality.

WHY IT WORKS   The heart of this program is mind over matter, which addresses the fundamental problem most overweight people have with dieting. They want to diet, they have a thousand reasons why they should, but when the time comes to make those critical food choices on a daily basis, they find themselves unable to do so. *Not Another Diet Book* offers a method to overcome that inability.

Although the author's theory and method of Reflective Relearning may be controversial, her advice about nutrition and exercise is sound. This book offers no biochemical shortcuts. Sommer clearly and persuasively discusses the shortcomings of many fad diets and diet therapies, such as injections, pills, and surgery. If you aren't yet convinced to stay clear of them, perhaps Sommer can save you some grief.

The book is written clearly and is easy to read. The case histories are interesting and provide insight, identification, and even comfort. Sommer's program is laid out in easily understood terms and the investment for anyone who tries this program is minimal: 10 minutes of your time per day for six weeks. The potential benefits are well worth it.

POTENTIAL DRAWBACKS   Some of Sommer's criticisms of popular diets may be overstated. She suggests, for example, that all diets are based upon the deprivation/reward system. This is not quite true. There are exceptions.

It is unlikely that Sommer's theory can be scientifically proved, and so we can only trust that her case histories are accurate. This creates something of a paradox: you must believe the program will work in order for it to have any chance of working, yet you cannot be sure it works unless you have already experienced positive results. Consequently, you must be willing to employ a bit of faith.

SECOND OPINION "This book helps the reader to understand the basics of inappropriate eating behaviors and outlines steps needed to change them."

—*Current Diet Review*

THE SETPOINT DIET

by Gilbert A. Leveille, Ph.D.
Ballantine Books
Clinton, Indiana: 1985

ABOUT THE AUTHOR   A graduate of Rutgers University who holds a Ph.D. in nutrition and biochemistry, Dr. Leveille was chairman of the department of food sciences and human nutrition at Michigan State University for 10 years. He is also a former president of the Institute of Food Technology and of the National Nutrition Consortium, and a former chair of the Food and Nutrition Board of the National Research Council of the National Academy of Sciences. He lectures widely and has published over 300 scientific papers. The fundamentals of this diet are based on research Leveille conducted during his three years as director of nutrition and health science at General Foods Corporation.

WHOM IT'S FOR   *The Setpoint Diet* is for almost anyone with any amount of weight to lose, from teenagers (girls 15 or older, boys 16 or older) to the elderly (up to age 80). Exceptions are pregnant women, nursing mothers, and anyone with a serious illness.

OVERVIEW   According to Leveille's research findings, the body has a setpoint, a weight it will maintain—and, in a sense, *defend*—regardless of caloric intake (within reason). His theory suggests that many overweight people have a high setpoint, which makes losing weight very difficult. According to his theory, the only way to lose weight and keep it off is to lower the body's setpoint to match ideal body weight. The only known safe and effective way to do this is through moderate daily exercise. Thus, Leveille's plan has two major components: a moderate calorie reduction, allowing for nutritional balance and variation, and an exercise plan.

The nutritional plan focuses on creating daily menus by making guided choices from various food groups. Leveille groups foods together as follows:

Group one: breads, cereals, starchy foods

Group two: fruits

Group three: milk and other dairy products

Group four: meat, fish, poultry

Group five: vegetables

Bonus foods: special high-calorie foods and snack foods to be eaten in limited amounts

Freebie foods: noncaloric or very-low-calorie beverages and seasonings

Rather than prescribe specific calorie counting, *The Setpoint Diet* provides general menus based upon these groups and recommends portion sizes based upon the weight goal of the dieter.

The exercise plan is simple: a half hour per day of moderate exercise, such as a brisk walk, climbing stairs, raking leaves, mowing the lawn, waxing the floor. Whatever the exercise, it must be continuous for 30 minutes; golf, tennis, and other competitive sports thus do not work.

The program is outlined as follows:

Step one: Find your goal weight on the Mutual Life Insurance table.

Step two: Set a realistic weight loss schedule (usually between one and three pounds per week).

Step three: Begin an exercise program.

Step four: Calculate your daily caloric needs for your weight loss goal, based on Leveille's formula, then select the appropriate caloric level for your personal diet—1,200, 1,500, 1,800, 2,100, or 2,400 calories per day. Dieters over 65 may, with their physician's approval, go below 1,200 calories in order to meet their special needs, and teenaged dieters may eat more than 2,400.

Step five: Here begins the portion control program. Basic portion sizes are given for foods in each of the basic groups; portion sizes within each group are calorically equivalent. The diet is based upon a specified number of portions per meal per day. Exercise levels are maintained at a minimum of a half hour per day.

Leveille recommends that when dieters reach their ideal weight, they increase their caloric intake while maintaining the portion control of the diet and, if desired, decrease moderate aerobic exercise to three times per week, doing light exercise on the other days.

NUTRITIONAL EVALUATION   The caloric level of two days' average menus was above the 1,500 suggested by the author. Thus, a dieter on this program will need to be careful with portion sizes and perhaps decrease some slightly from what the diet recommends. Calories break down nutritionally as follows:

```
Carbohydrates ........................... 46%
Protein ................................. 23%
Fat ..................................... 31%
Sodium .................................. 2,950 milligrams
Fiber ................................... 18 grams
Cholesterol ............................. 257 milligrams
```

ANALYSIS OF 2-DAY MENU FOR FEMALE, AGE 35

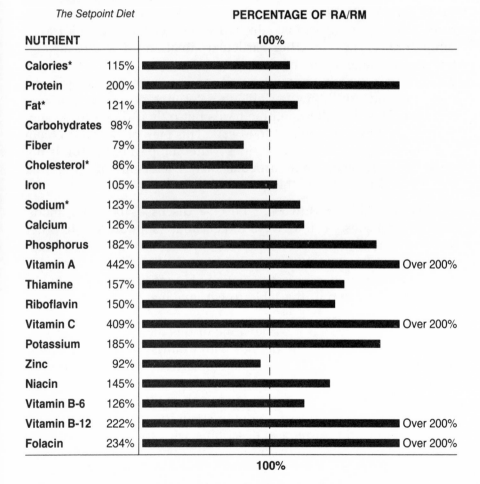

NUTRIENT		PERCENTAGE OF RA/RM
The Setpoint Diet		**100%**
Calories*	115%	
Protein	200%	
Fat*	121%	
Carbohydrates	98%	
Fiber	79%	
Cholesterol*	86%	
Iron	105%	
Sodium*	123%	
Calcium	126%	
Phosphorus	182%	
Vitamin A	442%	Over 200%
Thiamine	157%	
Riboflavin	150%	
Vitamin C	409%	Over 200%
Potassium	185%	
Zinc	92%	
Niacin	145%	
Vitamin B-6	126%	
Vitamin B-12	222%	Over 200%
Folacin	234%	Over 200%

100%

*Recommended maximum allowance. Nutrient should not exceed 100%.

Protein is too high, though it would be acceptable if the carbohydrates were at least 55 percent. Overall, these percentages are not as good as the other weight loss books I have analyzed. Carbohydrates are low, even by the pre-1989 goals in effect when the book was written. Cholesterol is within recommended goals, but dietary fat is above the upper guideline limits. By replacing the whole milk in this diet with skim or nonfat milk and milk products, the dieter can reduce both cholesterol and dietary fat. Sodium is higher than recommended.

The diet meets 100 percent of the RDA for all essential vitamins and minerals except for zinc, which is above two-thirds of the RDA.

PRACTICALITY   This diet is very flexible. The three meals and three snacks per day can be adjusted when necessary to suit travel, dining out, parties, or other particular situations. The diet also allows moderate amounts of alcohol and desserts. Dieters do have to plan meals to some degree in advance, however, and weigh and measure foods until they feel able to determine proper portion size on sight. This diet allows ethnic foods but only if they can be substituted for those on the diet food lists. This may present a problem for some of the more exotic cuisines—after all, part of the fun is not quite knowing what's in a particular dish. Dieters are also required to keep food records, another potential inconvenience.

LIFESTYLE AND EXERCISE   Leveille discusses behavior modification strategies, such as ways to get family support, create other support systems, and achieve portion control through record keeping, along with ways to prevent boredom and other emotions that commonly threaten successful dieting. He stresses eating slowly, always sitting down at the table to eat, making meals special, and avoiding hasty food choices.

Aerobic exercise is a cornerstone of this diet. Leveille suggests rigorous activity (which he defines with examples) for half an hour five times a week, and a lighter aerobic activity (also defined with examples) the other two days. This, according to Leveille, is the minimum amount of exercise needed to change the body's setpoint.

The Setpoint Diet goes into depth about the theory and practice of safe and healthful exercise, describing why and how it works as well as offering tips on warm-up, cool-down, and how to know when you've overdone it.

WHY IT WORKS   *The Setpoint Diet* is a sensible approach to weight loss, balancing moderate caloric restriction with exercise and behavior modification. Variety and flexibility within the food program can help prevent feelings of deprivation, and the emphasis on exercise gives the dieter a good chance of succeeding. Although Leveille's setpoint theory about body weight and exercise has never been empirically proved, many other weight loss benefits of exercise *have*: it burns calories, burns fat, speeds up the body's metabolic rate (for as much as two hours after a workout), builds lean muscle tissue, and even reduces appetite.

POTENTIAL DRAWBACKS   The record-keeping can be cumbersome and, at times, irritating for some people. Also, dieters who, for medical or other reasons, have to be on a fat-restricted diet will need to alter some of the recipes that call for whole-milk dairy products.

SECOND OPINION   *"The Setpoint Diet* by Dr. Gilbert Leveille offers a refreshingly accurate and realistic approach to weight management."

—*Current Diet Review*

THE STOP-LIGHT DIET
FOR CHILDREN

by Leonard H. Epstein, Ph.D., and
Sally Squires, M.S.
Little Brown and Company
New York: 1988

ABOUT THE AUTHORS   Dr. Epstein is a psychologist and clinical professor of psychiatry at the University of Pittsburgh. Sally Squires is a medical writer for the *Washington Post*. She has won the Psychiatric Institute Foundation's Mental Health Achievement Award along with other journalistic awards in the area of psychology.

WHOM IT'S FOR   This program is designed for 6- to 12-year-olds who weigh at least 20 percent above the national average for their age, height, and sex, although it can be successfully applied to children who are as little as 10 percent overweight. The Stop-Light Diet is *not* recommended for children who are only a few pounds overweight; such children should probably not be put on a weight loss diet of any kind. Nor is it for any child more than 50 percent above normal weight; such seriously obese children need the structured, multidisciplinary teaching of professionals.

OVERVIEW   This is a family-oriented diet to address a problem that involves the entire family. Its objective is to help parents and children work together to make a positive impact upon the overweight child's eating and exercise habits. It is geared toward gradual, safe weight loss based upon good food choices and sensible portion sizes. No foods are excluded, so that the child's feelings of deprivation do not sabotage success. The diet's philosophy is this: Parents should not have to force children to make huge sacrifices during the eight-week program or beyond. Weight loss is for a lifetime. If you control the food you consume, you stop letting the food control you.

Some chapters in the book are written for parents, others for children, with language appropriate for each to ensure the equal involvement of all parties. The diet is organized into eight weekly lessons about food and making the right meal choices.

To enable children to understand that not all foods were created equal and to educate them about which foods are good for them and which are not, *The Stop-Light Diet* groups foods according to colors, using the familiar image of the traffic signal to illustrate: green foods are the best, yellow foods are good, red foods are not good. The authors provide comprehensive lists of the foods that fall into each of these three categories. They support their designations with data about nutrient density (the nutritional value per calorie of a given food). The authors instruct parents to buy red, yellow, and green stickers and color-code all the food in the house so that children can make informed choices and begin to understand the benefits and consequences of those choices.

The authors recommend caloric levels of between 900 and 1,200 per day, depending on height, weight, age, and activity level. Their eight-week program is presented as follows:

Week one: Learn the stoplight signals

Week two: Learn the ABCs of smart eating

Week three: Praise and privileges

Week four: Time to exercise

Week five: Set a good example (for your parents)

Week six: Keep to the stoplight signals

Week seven: Remember the rules

Week eight: Stay trim and healthy forever

The book encourages parents to set good examples in their own food choices and to set up food diaries for themselves and for their children in order to make monitoring diet a family activity. The program outlines a system of praise and rewards so that parents and child share a structure of positive reinforcement.

The book addresses the issue of biological hunger versus psychological hunger, making the point that the latter can be relieved without food. The authors also describe the importance of aerobic exercise as a part of a child's lifestyle. They point out the child's need for a support system and suggest ways to set one up.

NUTRITIONAL EVALUATION   A sample day's meal plan found the calories almost 150 below the book's own recommendations. Those calories break down as follows:

Carbohydrates 60%
Protein 23%
Fat 17%
Sodium .... 1,676 milligrams
Fiber .... 18 grams
Cholesterol .... 71 milligrams

ANALYSIS OF 1-DAY MENU FOR MALE, AGE 6

The Stop-Light Diet for Children

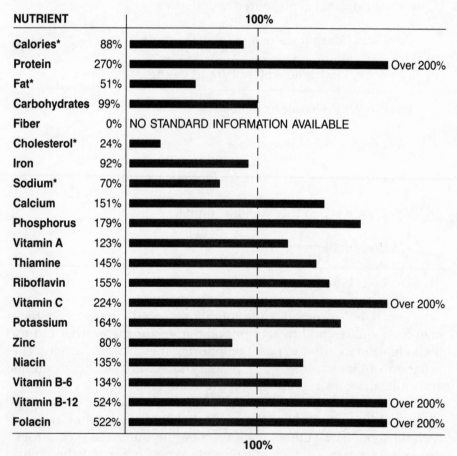

PERCENTAGE OF RA/RM

NUTRIENT		100%
Calories*	88%	
Protein	270%	Over 200%
Fat*	51%	
Carbohydrates	99%	
Fiber	0%	NO STANDARD INFORMATION AVAILABLE
Cholesterol*	24%	
Iron	92%	
Sodium*	70%	
Calcium	151%	
Phosphorus	179%	
Vitamin A	123%	
Thiamine	145%	
Riboflavin	155%	
Vitamin C	224%	Over 200%
Potassium	164%	
Zinc	80%	
Niacin	135%	
Vitamin B-6	134%	
Vitamin B-12	524%	Over 200%
Folacin	522%	Over 200%

100%

*Recommended maximum allowance. Nutrient should not exceed 100%.

Protein is slightly higher than recommended goals—even the more liberal pre-1989 goals—but at a level I would still consider acceptable for a children's diet, especially since fat and carbohydrates both fall within the goals. Fiber is a little low according to adult standards, but there are no fiber standards available for children.

All essential vitamins and minerals meet at least 100 percent of the RDA except for iron and zinc, which are well above two-thirds of the RDA.

PRACTICALITY   *The Stop-Light Diet* is, for the most part, geared to the realities of family life. It contains a number of wise suggestions, such as how to replace traditional candy and other food rewards with nonfattening alternatives, as well as some practical advice on how to thwart well-meaning but sabotaging friends, relatives, and even school lunch programs. Parents can also benefit from the nutritional information and the authors' recommendations, and they may find that setting a good example for their children is the best thing they ever did for themselves.

The program requires a serious commitment from both parents and children, and some aspects can be time-consuming—particularly the need for every member of the family to count his or her own caloric intake, measuring and weighing foods, and recording all of his. Helping a child learn about nutrition is not done in one sitting, and for busy working parents this may create time conflicts. But this minor sacrifice is worthwhile when a child's health and future are at stake.

LIFESTYLE AND EXERCISE   The book presents what may be the most effective behavioral modification technique: learning by example. This is both an opportunity and a responsibility for parents. The authors also present a number of other methods for transforming a child's behavior: a habit book, parent/child contracts, cue control, TV-viewing limits, and other rule setting, to name a few. The program urges parents to set realistic expectations and to work with the child for gradual change. Old habits die hard. In this respect, children can be thankful that their habits are relatively new.

The Stop-Light Diet offers a comprehensive approach to helping an inactive child become (and *want* to become) active. The authors' tips and insights (including a well-defined exercise/calorie expenditure chart) help make the issue of exercise concrete, and therefore accessible, to children.

WHY IT WORKS   The Stop-Light Diet is based on scientific research from the Western Psychiatric Institute and Clinic and the University of Pittsburgh School of Medicine; it applies those research findings to promote safe, gradual weight loss not only for children but for the entire family. Its behavioral modification aspects are strong, showing parents not only how to instruct but also how to be coach, cheerleader, and role model (effective parenting techniques no matter what the specific objective).

But the book is not just about how parents can better guide their children toward weight control and a healthier life. This book speaks directly to overweight children and does so in a simple yet effective way, presenting information about nutrition, exercise, and behavior in a way that is meaningful to the child.

The high-fiber, low-fat diet combined with aerobic activity should become a part of the child's lifestyle. If so, it will make for a more healthful and satisfying childhood, adolescence, and adulthood.

POTENTIAL DRAWBACKS   The authors suggest daily weigh-ins, which can lead to frustration, especially on the part of a child who is unlikely to comprehend the nonlinear manner in which most people lose weight. At the very least, the child can experience unnecessary pressure from such constant monitoring of results.

Some of the nutritional information is overstated. The authors, for example, assert that skim milk has "significantly" more calcium than whole milk. In fact, the difference is only about 4 percent. Skim milk is, however, a more healthful choice for an overweight child, primarily because it has almost no fat, so that the overstatement, while erroneous, is not harmful.

Finally, this program requires a serious commitment on the part of parents. It would be nice but naive to believe that all parents are capable of this. Those who are not would do better to enroll their overweight child in a program that provides an external structure along with the family support.

SECOND OPINIONS   "The diet is based on sound nutritional advice and can be used by adults as well. As diet books go, it appears to be a worthwhile purchase."

—*Library Journal*

"Parents who seek a safe, effective diet for their overweight children will find much guidance here."

—*Publishers Weekly*

THE T-FACTOR DIET
by Martin Katahn, Ph.D.
W. W. Norton & Company
New York: 1989

ABOUT THE AUTHOR   Dr. Katahn holds a Ph.D. in psychology and is director of the weight management program at Vanderbilt University.

WHOM IT'S FOR   *The T-Factor Diet* is for any overweight individual looking for a safe, sane, and self-monitored lifelong approach to weight control. The book provides a modified program for children and adolescents.

OVERVIEW   The T-Factor Diet is based upon the concept of *thermogenesis*—the production of heat, especially in the body—and the widely recognized and generally accepted nutritional finding that the food group most influential in weight gain is fat.

According to Katahn, calories were *not* created equal. "You can't get fat except by eating fat!" The reason most overweight people are overweight, he says, is that they eat "four to five times more fat than is essential and about twice as much as is necessary to make a tasty, healthy, lifelong weight-maintenance diet."

Katahn goes into considerable detail to support these claims, describing such aspects as:

- The thermic effect of food: the body uses differing numbers of calories to convert various kinds of foods—protein, carbohydrates, fat—into usable energy.

- Adaptive thermogenesis: the ability of the body to adapt to changing circumstances by conserving or wasting calories.

- The body's fat storage process: four parts fat to one part water, so that when weight loss is due to the loss of water, very little fat is shed.

- The thermic effect of exercise: how substantial, repetitive movements used up stored fat.

Katahn suggests that total caloric intake is not a key issue in weight control. Rather, total *fat* intake determines total bodily fat. Conversely, a diet high in complex carbohydrates, Katahn suggests, will raise the body's metabolism and precipitate weight loss and weight control. Of course, too much of any food can hinder weight loss in some people, and the author tempers his claim by offering two forms of the T-Factor Diet: one in which calories as well as total dietary fat are counted; one in which they are not.

The T-Factor formula for weight loss is simple:

- For women, a maximum of 20 to 40 grams of fat per day.

- For men, a maximum of 30 to 60 grams of fat per day.

Even at the high end of this formula, most people will be cutting their present fat intake in half. The dieter is allowed to compensate for the reduced fat with whatever increase in complex carbohydrates is needed in order to satisfy the appetite.

In addition to this formula, the author provides suggestions for basic low-fat breakfasts, lunches, and dinners, as well as three weeks of daily menus for those who feel the need for a specific eating plan.

Katahn lists low-fat substitutes for common high-fat foods and offers general fat-cutting tips and low-fat recipes. He makes the important distinction between bad fats (saturated) and good fats (poly- and monounsaturated) and discusses the importance of dietary fiber to the body-fat equation and to general good health.

Katahn emphasizes the importance of dietary variety, warning against any kind of food obsession. He illustrates the effectiveness of his program by describing his own weight control experiences on it.

He predicts that dieters on his program of low-fat eating and aerobic exercise can lose one to one and a half pounds per week but recognizes that some people may be exceptions. For them, or for anyone wishing to lose weight faster, he offers the Quick Melt plan, a low-fat *and* calorie-restricted plan.

According to Katahn, the combination of low fats and calorie restriction accelerates the rate at which the body pulls fat from fat cells. Quick Melt's caloric levels range from 1,000 to 1,300 for women, and 1,500 to 1,800 for men. He predicts a fairly rapid weight loss that will depend on the total amount of weight the individual needs to lose: the more overweight the person, the faster the initial weight comes off. The Quick Melt program offers three weeks of menus. Katahn recommends taking a multiple vitamin and mineral each day to ensure adequate nutrition at the moderately low caloric levels.

For those who choose to go on the Quick Melt plan, it is advisable to switch back to the core program after every three weeks in order to reduce the potential stress often associated with reduced caloric intake.

Maintenance on the regular (non-calorie-restricted) T-Factor Diet is literally just that: maintaining the same low consumption of dietary fat. For those on the Quick Melt plan, maintenance begins with a transition period during which the dieter increases protein and carbohydrate calories, maintaining low fat levels, until he or she reaches a comfortable total caloric level.

Katahn has created a modified version of the T-Factor Diet for children and adolescents. He does not recommend that they count calories or fat grams. Rather, he urges that parents provide a healthy eating environment at home, permit the child's appetite to determine his or her food intake, and provide nutritious and good-tasting meals and snacks at every opportunity. The program suggests ways to deal with various eating situations, including fast-food restaurants. Katahn suggests tips for getting an overweight child or teen to exercise and also offers prudent advice about allowing a slightly overweight child to grow into his or her body weight. Finally, Katahn provides suggestions for people who want better health and weight management without weight loss.

NUTRITIONAL EVALUATION   I looked at a two-day average from the regular T-Factor Diet and from the Quick Melt menus designed for more rapid weight loss. On the regular diet, the calories were within an acceptable range (the author makes no specific caloric recommendations). Those calories break down as follows:

```
Carbohydrates ........................... 59%
Protein ................................. 27%
Fat ..................................... 14%
Sodium .................................. 1,697 milligrams
Fiber ................................... 20 grams
Cholesterol ............................. 246 milligrams
```

Protein is too high, and I would suggest that anyone on this diet reduce protein intake along with counting fat grams. The rest of the numbers are all within recommended goals. All essential vitamins and minerals meet 100 percent of the RDA except for iron, which is above two-thirds of the RDA.

ANALYSIS OF 2-DAY MENU FOR FEMALE, AGE 35

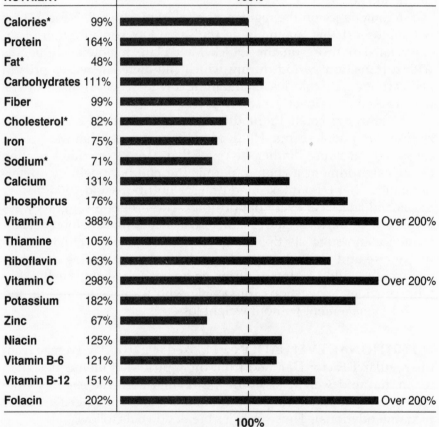

The T-Factor Diet

PERCENTAGE OF RA/RM

NUTRIENT		100%
Calories*	99%	
Protein	164%	
Fat*	48%	
Carbohydrates	111%	
Fiber	99%	
Cholesterol*	82%	
Iron	75%	
Sodium*	71%	
Calcium	131%	
Phosphorus	176%	
Vitamin A	388%	Over 200%
Thiamine	105%	
Riboflavin	163%	
Vitamin C	298%	Over 200%
Potassium	182%	
Zinc	67%	
Niacin	125%	
Vitamin B-6	121%	
Vitamin B-12	151%	
Folacin	202%	Over 200%

100%

*Recommended maximum allowance. Nutrient should not exceed 100%.

Two days on the Quick Melt menus averaged to an acceptable caloric range, broken down as follows:

Carbohydrates 62%
Protein 25%
Fat 13%
Sodium .... 1,225 milligrams
Fiber .... 19 grams
Cholesterol .... 136 milligrams

ANALYSIS OF 2-DAY MENU FOR FEMALE, AGE 35

The T-Factor Quick Melt Diet

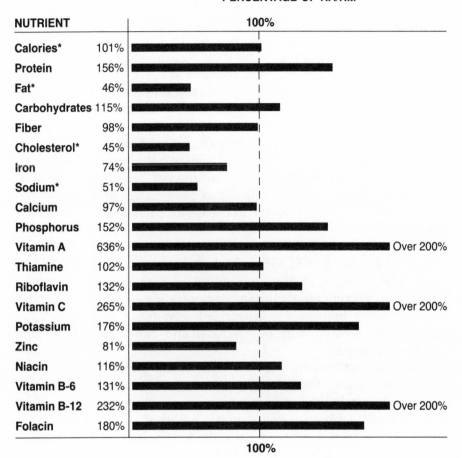

PERCENTAGE OF RA/RM

NUTRIENT		100%
Calories*	101%	
Protein	156%	
Fat*	46%	
Carbohydrates	115%	
Fiber	98%	
Cholesterol*	45%	
Iron	74%	
Sodium*	51%	
Calcium	97%	
Phosphorus	152%	
Vitamin A	636%	Over 200%
Thiamine	102%	
Riboflavin	132%	
Vitamin C	265%	Over 200%
Potassium	176%	
Zinc	81%	
Niacin	116%	
Vitamin B-6	131%	
Vitamin B-12	232%	Over 200%
Folacin	180%	

100%

*Recommended maximum allowance. Nutrient should not exceed 100%.

Protein is high and fiber is a bit low, which is surprising given the relatively high percentage of carbohydrates. All the other numbers fall within recommended goals. All essential vitamins and minerals meet 100 percent of the RDA except for iron, calcium, and zinc, which are all above two-thirds of the RDA.

PRACTICALITY Thanks to a growing awareness on the part of the American public and the accommodations of some food manufacturers and restaurants, low-fat eating presents little practical or logistical difficulty for most people. *The T-Factor Diet* presents information about hidden fats that can help offset the deceptive practices of some food providers. The absence of any rigid food substitutions makes most eating situations easy to manage, and the universality of the principles—the fact that low-fat eating is a key not only to weight management but to overall health—means that the entire family can participate, providing they are convinced of the benefits of doing so. Although the diet requires keeping track of daily fat grams, this should be less taxing than calorie calculations.

Although the Quick Melt plan requires calorie counting, it is, for that kind of program, relatively flexible and easy to implement. The transitional phase to maintenance is particularly sensible, with menus that ensure proper nutrition and an eating plan to suit individual needs. The recipes include nutritional information on cholesterol, fat, dietary fiber, sodium, and calories for informed eating; this makes caloric calculations on the Quick Melt a relatively simple matter.

LIFESTYLE AND EXERCISE   The behavioral emphasis of this program is on avoiding deprivation, adopting a healthy way of eating rather than putting yourself in a temporary state of hunger. Katahn suggests ways to prevent hunger between meals and to achieve satisfaction through attitude changes and nutritious and filling snacks and meals.

Katahn outlines the "T-Factor fat burning exercise program," first by describing the differences between anaerobic and aerobic exercise. Anaerobic exercise (in which activity stops and starts often) burns mostly carbohydrates; aerobic (continuous) exercise burns mostly fat. Katahn then gives his picks for the best aerobic exercise and suggests the best ways to do it. He addresses such issues as training heart rate and endurance, the best times of day to exercise, as well as variances in duration and intensity level. He warns, for example, that an increase in duration and intensity may lead to a slight temporary weight gain because increased activity can cause muscles to take up extra glycogen from the next meal; glycogen (a form of converted carbohydrate, stored in the liver and the muscles) retains water.

The T-Factor Diet addresses the unique fat-burning problems of swimming as an aerobic exercise. It also covers the psychological aspects of exercise, such as how it can enhance self-esteem, and the importance of setting realistic exercise expectations.

WHY IT WORKS   *The T-Factor Diet* is easy to read and understand, and you can begin its program virtually immediately. The diet is based on sound, scientifically verifiable data. Because the diet is also designed to benefit general health, most people who follow it should discover that they feel better. This is a tremendous incentive to stick with it. There are no known negative side effects.

Katahn warns the reader against diet soft drinks and other artificially sweetened products, which, he believes, only serve to perpetuate a sweet tooth and increase hunger. In general, he seems to have a deep understanding of the potential pitfalls of any weight control program and offers some sensible ways to assuage them.

His discussion of hidden fats is educational and helpful to anyone determined to follow a low-fat diet in a world littered with high-fat land mines. Katahn's stories about his own weight loss experiences are inspirational, enlightening, and reassuring. His advice to restrict weighing-in to a minimum is wise.

POTENTIAL DRAWBACKS   The lifestyle section is brief and the advice may be overly simplistic, such as the counsel to "just avoid" problems that may lead to high-fat eating. Many dieters would, therefore, need to supplement this diet with a more profound approach to transcending the emotional and behavioral issues linked to excess weight.

Some of the dietary recommendations—such as *no fried foods ever*—may be extreme for most people and do not reflect the voice of moderation that is characteristic of the rest of the program.

Finally, the author claims to be presenting breakthrough information when in fact his program is based upon widely known and understood data. This, in fact, is one of the program's strengths, but the author's claim to innovation seems a bit exaggerated.

SECOND OPINION   *"The T-Factor Diet* is recommended for readers who are highly motivated to begin following a low-fat diet plan! The reader is cautioned about the lack of behavioral modification guidelines."

—*Current Diet Review*

WINNING WEIGHT LOSS
FOR TEENS
by Joanne Ikeda, M.A., R.D.
Bull Publishing Company
Palo Alto, California: 1987

ABOUT THE AUTHOR Ikeda is a nutrition specialist at the University of California at Berkeley Cooperative Extension.

WHOM IT'S FOR As the title suggests, this book is aimed at overweight teenagers, but it is also for their parents so that they can provide encouragement and support.

OVERVIEW This book begins by distinguishing itself from a traditional diet. *Winning Weight Loss for Teens* instead describes itself as an approach to "changing bad food and activity habits." Ikeda promises the teenager rewards for making those changes: more energy and better-looking skin, in addition to the obviously more attractive body. The author encloses a contract for the teenager to sign, initiating his or her commitment to this program.

The program begins with a review of current habits. Ikeda suggests that the teenager make a food diary, and she gives instructions for analyzing the results to pinpoint both good and bad current eating habits. With that as a starting point, Ikeda introduces the teenager to a healthful alternative, advising three meals and two snacks at regular times each day. She emphasizes setting small, reachable goals and suggests simple ways of adjusting the three-meal/two-snack approach to accommodate special circumstances.

Winning Weight Loss for Teens goes beyond what to eat; it addresses the equally important issue of *how* to eat, discussing the merits of slow eating and of drinking plenty of water.

The food diary remains a part of the program throughout, allowing the dieter to learn from his or her eating habits as they change. The author contends that the simple act of recording what is eaten reduces food intake by 10 percent. The diary, of which the book provides sample pages, is also for recording exercise and feelings, good or bad. Ikeda recommends setting realistic and attainable goals; she advises readers that it normally takes three to six months to change food habits and reach an ideal body weight.

The author explains the value of aerobic exercise and provides guidelines for getting started. She discusses the genetic realities of weight control, basic body types, metabolic rates, and the impact of caloric consumption on weight. She prescribes an approach to eating that can help virtually any teenager achieve weight control by cutting calories through nutritional awareness and intelligent food substitutions.

Ikeda creates a positive approach to weight maintenance. She begins by congratulating the teenager and ends with tips on how to adjust habits if the teenager starts to regain excess weight.

NUTRITIONAL EVALUATION Since there are no formal diet plan, menus, or recipes, nutrition will vary depending on the specific choices of the dieter. The diet does conform to the four basic food groups of U.S. dietary guidelines, and the kinds of food choices the diet emphasizes will encourage healthful nutrition.

PRACTICALITY The book is easy reading, with age-appropriate language in a breezy, non-preachy style, a clear format, and a workbook approach. The family orientation is not so demanding as to preclude participation by busy working parents—or active teenagers.

LIFESTYLE AND EXERCISE Behavioral modification is a large part of this program, beginning with the whole notion of self-monitoring and self-reflection on behavior. The author also makes some practical suggestions for coping with potentially difficult situations, such as holidays with their traditional heavy meals. She advises rehearsing potential conflicts ahead of time in order to prepare the best response. Without getting on any moral soapbox, Ikeda points out the caloric realities of alcohol as well as the appetite stimulation of marijuana. Many of her ideas about behavioral self-management are based upon her own published research (*Journal of Nutrition Education*, vol. 14, no. 3, 1982).

This program stresses aerobic exercise as an essential part of any successful approach to weight control. Suggestions and diagrams about time, frequency, kind of exercise, and warming up and cooling down are included. Organized sports need not be the focus.

WHY IT WORKS   The book's tone is positive and not condescending. I believe that many teenagers will be inspired to at least give the advice a try. With no specific food plan, this program celebrates individuality within the guidelines of what is healthy and nonfattening. This is particularly important to teenagers, for whom the implied authority of a rigid diet may be a complete turn-off. The general suggestions conform to U.S. dietary guidelines, and they encourage variety and nutrient density (the per-calorie nutritional value of a given food).

Rather than focus on food, the program concentrates the teenager's attention on self-esteem and behavior, providing a framework for gradual successes that foster the encouragement many teens need to succeed at weight control.

POTENTIAL DRAWBACKS   I found one conflicting suggestion, and a minor one at that: after recommending that teens find non-food rewards for themselves, Ikeda lists some examples—and includes lunch with a friend and a picnic.

Otherwise, the only potential shortcoming of this book is that it may be too "soft" for those teens for whom externally imposed structure with group support is necessary to achieve weight control. (I should point out that Ikeda has published a companion book, *Winning Weight Management for Teens: A How to Conduct a Weight Loss Program for Teens Manual*. It is designed to help registered dietitians or other health professionals create and conduct an organized weight loss program.)

SECOND OPINIONS   *"Winning Weight Loss for Teens* is a sound, practical guide to weight control for literate youth."

—*Journal of The American Dietetic Association*

"This book will be a valuable addition to any weight-management program for adolescents."

—*Journal of Nutrition Education*

WEIGHT-CONTROL DIETS

FOR THOSE WHO NEED TO GAIN WEIGHT

EATING TO *GAIN* WEIGHT IS AS serious a matter for some as losing weight is for others. In fact, many of the same rules apply. For example: just as a safe rate of weight loss is about one to two pounds per week, a safe rate of gaining is about one to two pounds per week.

The best diets to modify for weight gain are those based upon gradual weight loss through healthful food choices. The same choices, with increased protein and overall calories, can translate to healthful weight gain. From those weight-loss diet books I have reviewed, I would recommend the following to modify for weight gain: *The New American Diet, Living Lean by Choosing More, The T-Factor Diet*, and *The Choose to Lose Diet* (which you could retitle "Choose to Gain").

Increase protein up to 20 percent while maintaining a high carbohydrate intake (50 percent and up) and keeping fat intake below 30 percent. Increase overall calories by about 500 per day. If this does not lead to weight gain, increase caloric intake slowly until you start to put on one to two pounds per week.

Exercise is also very important to healthful weight gain. By engaging in weight-bearing exercise—such as weight lifting or lifting on weight machines, doing repetitive motions—and by eating moderately elevated calories and protein, you can be sure the weight you gain will be lean muscle and not fat.

SECTION TWO

MEDICAL/HEALTH/ SPECIALTY DIETS

MEDICAL/HEALTH/SPECIALTY DIETS

ONE OF THE MOST EXCITING aspects of the field of diet and nutrition is the increasing evidence linking disease—its causes, prevention, treatment, and cure—to the foods we eat. Diet can have a greater impact on more illnesses than was previously understood. For this reason, any book calling itself *Diets That Work* must include dietary guidelines and treatments for specific illnesses. Health is a key concern here, but weight loss—and sometimes weight gain—is usually part of that concern; thus many of these books can be considered weight loss books also.

In selecting the conditions I would address, I considered those illnesses most profoundly affected by diet and nutrition. I also took into account the breadth of available scientific research about nutritional approaches to each illness. AIDS, for example, is not included because research is still relatively new and, though diet is believed to be significant, specific recommendations could change radically in a brief span of time.

Of course, while the medical conditions addressed in this section have years of research behind them, breakthroughs may shed new light on them as well. For this reason, no dietary approach to an illness should be undertaken without the supervision of a physician. On the other hand, not all doctors are aware of all there is to know about the nutritional aspects of all illnesses. Thus, the insights in these books can be invaluable to you in managing some medical conditions and in working with your doctor.

Since diet books about managing a medical condition are obviously written for those who have the condition (and for their friends, relatives, and caregivers), the heading *Whom it's for* is no longer necessary. Other than that, the format in this section remains the same. Although exercise is not a factor in the effective management of all of these illnesses, it is important to many of them, and thus that heading is retained.

155

MEDICAL/HEALTH/SPECIALTY DIETS

ARTHRITIS

THIS IS A CATEGORY ENCOMPASSING over 100 diseases in which one or more joints are inflamed. Of these, three major types of arthritis have been found to respond favorably in varying degrees to dietary modifications:

1. *Rheumatoid arthritis*: The most common type and the most crippling (one in six sufferers develops deformities). It is an inflammation of the synovial membrane, the tissue within the joint.

2. *Osteoarthritis*: A degenerative condition that affects bones by breaking down their covering cartilage. Weight control is especially important in dealing with this condition.

3. *Gout*: In most cases, a hereditary disease that leads to an accumulation of uric acid crystals in the joints, particularly those of the foot, big toe, and thumb.

There is no known cure for arthritis. Even if the pain stops for long periods of time, the potential remains for reinflammation and future flare-ups. Arthritis sufferers commonly experience a worsening in their condition as the result of changes in barometric pressure, mental or physical stress, or reactions to specific "trigger" foods such as whole milk and organ meats.

One important dietary factor related to the treatment of arthritis concerns hormonelike substances produced by the body called prostaglandins, which play a primary role in the onset and relief of arthritis. The "bad" prostaglandins, linoleic and arachidonic acids, can bring on joint inflammation, while the "good" prostaglandin, eicosapentanoic (EPA) fish oil, has been found to decrease or even prevent flare-ups.

Although the body produces these substances, they can also be consumed in foods. Saturated fats, particularly from meat and poly-unsaturated fats have been found to contain the bad prostaglandins, while cold-water marine fish and marine plants contain the helpful EPA fish oil, which is also available as a nutritional supplement. Recent short-term studies have found beneficial results for arthritis sufferers who consume EPA capsules.

The following book explores these factors and the results of other dietary studies as potential ways of reducing the suffering of those with rheumatoid arthritis. (Most of today's dietary research has been collected in tests using rheumatoid arthritis sufferers. However, these dietary strategies may also prove beneficial for other types of arthritis patients.)

THE ARTHRITIS RELIEF DIET

by James Scala, Ph.D.
New American Library
New York: 1990

ABOUT THE AUTHOR   Dr. Scala has been involved in nutrition and health research for more than 20 years. A graduate of Cornell University with a doctoral degree in biochemistry, he has taught nutrition/biochemistry at Georgetown Medical School, the University of Oklahoma Medical School, Ohio College of Medicine, and the University of California at Berkeley. He is an elected member of the American Dietetic Association, the American Institute of Nutrition, the American College of Nutrition, and the British Nutrition Society. His previous books include *Eating Right for a Bad Gut* (see Inflammatory Bowel Disease section of this book) and *The High Blood Pressure Relief Diet*.

OVERVIEW   The author's goal is to help people with arthritis gain control of their health and regain the quality in their lives. Scala's research, which included a survey of folk remedies and a history of arthritis dating back to our Neanderthal ancestors, has led him to believe that dietary management of prostaglandins can help accomplish that goal. A careful diet supplemented with EPA fish oil, he believes, can be beneficial to those with arthritis. His five inflammation-fighting dietary strategies are as follows:

1. Change protein sources from high-fat meats to low-fat fish, poultry, skim milk and other low-fat dairy products, along with beans and vegetables; protein should comprise 10–15 percent of daily calories.

2. Reduce fat to 20–25 percent of daily calories, minimizing saturated fat and reducing polyunsaturated oils (which contain arachidonic and linoleic acids), while consuming one to two grams of EPA fish oil daily, either from fish or capsules.

3. Get 60–70 percent of daily calories from complex carbohydrates.

4. Consume 25–35 grams, or at least one ounce, of fiber per day either from food or from fiber supplements.

5. Balance nutrients and use vitamin and mineral supplements to ensure up to 100 percent of the RDA for all essential nutrients.

To help the reader implement these strategies, Scala lists foods to emphasize (such as cold-water marine fish), foods to avoid (such as whole eggs, organ meats, red meat, and deli cold cuts), foods to eat occasionally (such as vegetarian pizza with skim mozzarella cheese, and soft drinks), and foods to be cautious about (such as members of the nightshade family—tomatoes, potatoes, eggplant, and peppers—as well as dairy products). His discussion of menu planning includes tips for dining out and 74 recipes for muffins, cereal, fish, poultry, and game dishes, egg dishes, vegetable dishes, salads and dressings, fruit dishes, and desserts.

Scala advances two reasons why arthritis sufferers need vitamin and mineral supplements: (1) Because of pain and the stress it causes, they often do not eat as well as other people; and (2) Some arthritis medications can interfere with nutrient absorption. He then recommends specific supplementation to ensure adequate nutrition. While he admits the lack of empirical evidence that vitamin and mineral supplements make a pronounced difference for people with arthritis, he also points out the lack of hard evidence against this advice.

Beyond the basics of good nutrition and the benefits of prostaglandins, Scala also advises arthritis sufferers to maintain their ideal body weight. The pain of arthritis can often lead people to seek high-calorie comfort foods in excess and to withdraw from physical activity. Needless to say, this combination is a prescription for becoming overweight.

Scala cautions against fad diets, and demonstrates how the reader can set realistic weight loss goals and achieve them through variations on his overall dietary recommendations. He suggests aiming at a weight loss of from one to two pounds per week.

Since one of the potential complications of rheumatoid arthritis is ulcers, Scala suggests further dietary and lifestyle modifications for arthritis patients who develop them, including the further reduction of fat and the avoidance of aspirin. Because another potential complication is hypertension, the author discusses the sodium/ potassium balance—how the body needs to have more potassium than sodium—and suggests ways to accomplish this.

Scala's dietary recommendations address not only the minimizing of painful flare-ups and the containment of arthritis complications, but also the ramifications of arthritis medicines. Since aspirin is often prescribed for arthritis symptoms, the author describes some of the negative side effects of that drug and how to compensate for them. For example, Scala recommends up to 500 extra milligrams of vitamin C to offset the heartburn and gastric pain aspirin can cause. He also discusses the use of steroids as well as some potentially successful folk remedies, which have no known side effects.

Finally, Scala urges readers to seek support as they cope with this painful illness. He advises how to start and run a support group and how to find what he calls "mental nourishment." The book contains motivational success stories about people who have managed to live full and enjoyable lives after contracting arthritis.

NUTRITIONAL EVALUATION   Since the diet does not specify portion size, I used the standard dietary portion sizes. Given that, the caloric level was reasonable and the breakdown of the major nutrients was as follows:

```
Carbohydrates  . . . . . . . . . . . . . . . . . . . . . . . . . . . . 50%
Protein . . . . . . . . . . . . . . . . . . . . . . . . . . . . . . . . . . 20%
Fat  . . . . . . . . . . . . . . . . . . . . . . . . . . . . . . . . . . . . . 30%
Sodium  . . . . . . . . . . . . . . . . . . . . . . . . . . . . . . . . . 2,170 milligrams
Fiber  . . . . . . . . . . . . . . . . . . . . . . . . . . . . . . . . . . . 21 grams
Cholesterol  . . . . . . . . . . . . . . . . . . . . . . . . . . . . . 407 milligrams
```

Fat, sodium, and fiber are all within recognized health guidelines. Protein falls within the pre-1989 guidelines, but carbohydrates are below pre-1989 as well as current recommended minimums. Cholesterol is high, but much of it comes from deep-water fish. These fish are high in EPA fish oil, which has been found to have a cholesterol-lowering effect. It should also be noted that though the fat percentage is at the 30 percent ceiling of all recommended guidelines, this diet is very low in saturated fat.

All essential micronutrients meet 100 percent of the RDA guidelines except for vitamin B-12, niacin, and zinc, which meet at least two-thirds of those guidelines. The author recommends the use of a multiple vitamin and mineral supplement, which should ensure 100 percent of all essential micronutrients.

ANALYSIS OF 1-DAY MENU FOR MALE, AGE 36

The Arthritis Relief Diet

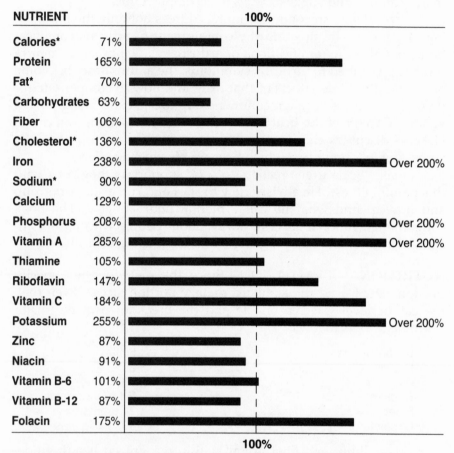

PERCENTAGE OF RA/RM

NUTRIENT		100%
Calories*	71%	
Protein	165%	
Fat*	70%	
Carbohydrates	63%	
Fiber	106%	
Cholesterol*	136%	
Iron	238%	Over 200%
Sodium*	90%	
Calcium	129%	
Phosphorus	208%	Over 200%
Vitamin A	285%	Over 200%
Thiamine	105%	
Riboflavin	147%	
Vitamin C	184%	
Potassium	255%	Over 200%
Zinc	87%	
Niacin	91%	
Vitamin B-6	101%	
Vitamin B-12	87%	
Folacin	175%	

100%

*Recommended maximum allowance. Nutrient should not exceed 100%.

PRACTICALITY   To accompany his EPA fish oil recommendations, Scala provides useful lists of types of fish and their EPA and polyunsaturated fat content. He also explains how to select cuts of fish with the highest EPA content.

The entire family can follow this book's food plan with favorable results, and the recipes range from easy-to-prepare to more complex for gourmets.

The book is thorough, addressing a wide range of problems facing people with arthritis. Scala even has advice for people who are sufficiently overweight to require liquid diets, so that they, too, can benefit from the research data on diet and its effects on reducing arthritis inflammation and pain. The style is clear and readable; each chapter ends with a helpful brief recap of its important points.

LIFESTYLE AND EXERCISE   Scala devotes a good deal of attention to the behavioral aspects of managing arthritis through dietary and lifestyle modifications. He recommends a food diary to help you get in touch with your body and its reactions to food, describing how to record your body's responses to various foods and drinks and how to interpret and make changes based upon those responses. He discusses techniques for label reading and demonstrates how to make careful food choices based upon your newfound knowledge and insight.

To help reduce the anxiety and depression often associated with arthritis, Scala recommends ways to maintain a proper blood-sugar level and suggests eliminating caffeine and alcohol.

Scala recognizes the need for arthritis sufferers to assume personal responsibility for themselves and offers methods for externalizing goals. For example, if your goal is losing weight, he suggests a "fat bag"—a bag of sand—along with an empty bag. Every time you lose weight, transfer an equivalent amount of sand from the full bag to the empty one.

Finally, he urges people with arthritis to make use of support groups, to learn coping techniques, and to set the goal of being a positive example for others.

Scala discusses the benefits of physical activity in terms of overall health as well as arthritis. Exercise, for example, can help in the restoration of damaged tissue by improving blood circulation, increasing flexibility, and preserving joint mobility. Also, increased oxygen to the brain can mean improved mental alertness, less depression as a result of the production of mood-elevating endorphins, and reduced vulnerability to emotional stress. Finally, exercise enhances bone strength and helps maintain weight to improve appearance and self-esteem. Scala recommends starting with a minimum of 15 minutes of exercise twice a day. He includes a good motivational pitch for why you should start immediately, citing the success of his 80-year-old mother who pedals her stationary cycle for 20 to 30 minutes per day. He gives some basic limbering, stretching, and breathing exercises and cautions against excessive physical exertion.

WHY IT WORKS   *The Arthritis Relief Diet* shows you how to reduce the foods and other lifestyle elements that cause arthritis flare-ups and how to increase those that moderate the flare-ups. The diet built around fish high in EPA and foods low in arachidonic and linoleic acids has been found to be beneficial in reducing the pain of arthritis. Scala shows readers simple ways to apply this research data to make a difference in their lives. He is thorough in his discourse—making it clear, for example, that fast-food fish does not promote arthritis relief and in fact may have the opposite effect. He tells the reader not only how to make the right food choices but also how to cook that food.

Scala provides both scientific and anecdotal information about arthritis management and makes clear which is which. The folk remedies he mentions, while not backed by scientific research, are interesting and may be useful to some people—provided they understand their speculative nature.

Scala's advice about nutritional supplements is pragmatic and thorough, giving the reader the necessary information to make an informed decision.

In general, the diet recommends the avoidance of chemical preservatives as much as possible. Such caution and focus on natural foods is good not only for arthritis relief but for overall good health.

Finally, unlike many of the books I have reviewed, this one does not make the mistake of listing mollusks (clams, oysters, and scallops) as high-cholesterol seafoods; they contain no more cholesterol than do fish, and Scala correctly reports this.

POTENTIAL DRAWBACKS My criticisms of this book are relatively minor. Scala recommends the avoidance of red meat and the dark meat of fowl in order to reduce saturated fat, then suggests the use of butter in cooking. He is inaccurate when he draws a direct connection between excess refined sugar and heart disease and when he reports the RDA for vitamin C at 65 milligrams (it is actually 60).

Otherwise, this book should be beneficial to those people with arthritis who are looking for a program of pain management that will also promote overall good health.

SECOND OPINION "While there is yet no definitive evidence that the proffered low-fat, low-cholesterol, high-fiber foods will fight inflammation, they are conducive to weight loss, which *is* known to help some arthritics."

—*Publishers Weekly*

MEDICAL/HEALTH/SPECIALTY DIETS

CALCIUM ABSORPTION

OVER TIME, LACK OF CALCIUM intake can lead to osteoporosis, a debilitating disease in which bones become porous and can easily break, fracture, or collapse, as is the case with the telltale "dowager's hump." Although osteoporosis is most common in women between the ages of 50 and 70 (one in four women of that age is afflicted), men over 50 are also at risk (one in eight suffers osteoporosis).

Prevention of this potentially crippling illness begins much earlier in life. While osteoporosis can result from genetic abnormalities or from being bedridden or wheelchair-bound and thus immobilized, the most common cause is a deficiency of dietary calcium over a period of years. The disease can begin—and be prevented—as early as age 20. For this reason, it is never too early to be concerned about calcium. The first book in this section addresses this concern.

Osteoporosis is not the only illness that involves calcium. Researchers have found a connection between calcium deficiencies and cancer, chiefly breast cancer.

Like all nutrients, calcium is only beneficial to the extent the body can absorb it. Consuming otherwise adequate amounts of calcium may not be enough if the *kind* of calcium is inadequate or if your body for some reason fails to absorb it correctly. The second book in this section presents an approach to the problem of calcium malabsorption.

Osteoporosis: Brittle Bones and the Calcium Crisis

by Kathleen Mayes
Pennant Books
Santa Barbara, California: 1986

ABOUT THE AUTHOR Kathleen Mayes is a free-lance medical writer who has done volunteer work for the American Heart Association and has more than 10 years' experience working with scriptwriters at the British Broadcasting Corporation. She is also author of *The Sodium-Watcher's Guide: Easy Ways to Cut Salt and Sodium*. She has done extensive research in the area of osteoporosis.

OVERVIEW The book begins with a sobering suggestion: because of our advanced technology, many of us will live longer than ever—but longer is not necessarily better if it includes the pain of osteoporosis. The author makes it clear that for most people this crippling illness is preventable and that prevention begins with a knowledge and understanding of the disease.

Mayes gives a detailed analysis of the cause, effects, symptoms, and potential dangers of osteoporosis. The book discusses early diagnosis as a part of prevention, recommending height measurements—and the recording of any height loss—as a part of routine medical examinations along with a close monitoring of skin thickness, since the thickness of skin often correlates to bone mass. Gum disease can also be an advance warning of osteoporosis. The author also suggests periodic CAT scans and other diagnostic procedures to ensure early detection of bone-mass loss.

The book provides an overview of the various bodily agents that play a role in bone growth, including growth hormones produced from the pituitary gland, thyroid hormones such as calcitonin and parathyroid hormones, sex hormones, and vitamin D. These agents ensure that the body maintains sufficient calcium in the bloodstream by stimulating calcium excretion from bone reserves, while at the same time replacing the calcium for storage in the bones. The author demonstrates how calcium consumption is only part of the osteoposis prevention equation. She discusses risk factors that are controllable, such as a diet low in calcium and other essential minerals, excessive alcohol consumption, cigarette smoking, and lack of weight-bearing exercise; along with those that are not controllable, such as family history.

This sets the stage for the thrust of the book: how to reduce risks of osteoporosis through changes in diet and lifestyle. Mayes provides guidelines for creating a regimen that can greatly reduce bone-mass loss.

She begins with a dietary focus on getting enough calcium and other important minerals and enabling the body to properly absorb those minerals. She points out that many Americans eat twice as much protein as is necessary; protein promotes calcium loss. Excess sodium, soft drinks, and coffee can also be "calcium blockers." The author recommends ways of eliminating these substances. Too much of a good thing—namely excess dietary fiber and protein—can also block calcium absorption; the author advises how much is too much. She suggests how much milk and milk products various individuals should consume (pregnant and postmenopausal women need more than others), the best low- and nonfat sources, and worthwhile calcium supplements.

Bone mass is an issue involving the entire lifestyle, so the author also points out that alcohol, street drugs, and many prescription medications can be calcium blockers and that stress depletes calcium. She discusses the safe use of medications that minimize calcium loss and also the pros and cons of estrogen and other hormones as treatment and prevention of osteoporosis.

She addresses the issues of airborne pollutants and their impact on calcium absorption and depletion. Inside the body, lead and other pollutants replace—and thus obliterate—calcium. Preventing osteoporosis includes reducing the lead in your immediate environment—for example, making sure not to use lead-based wall paints—while also doing whatever you can to breathe the cleanest air and drink the least polluted water.

Finally, Mayes discusses weight-bearing exercise, the kind that helps prevent and control osteoporosis.

You might say that the name of the osteoporosis prevention game is mineral management. This book outlines a plan of action to achieve just that.

NUTRITIONAL EVALUATION Although the book contains no recipes or menus, the foods most highly recommended will almost certainly ensure 100 percent of the RDA for calcium, magnesium, vitamin D, and the various other nutrients that play a role in maintaining bone mass.

PRACTICALITY This book organizes a good deal of complex and complicated information into a clearly written source of valuable tips and guidelines. Most of the advice is easy to follow. The beginning of the book should be motivational for many people.

One puzzling recommendation, however, is to read nutritional labels to determine the phosphorus-to-calcium ratio of foods—phosphorus is not commonly listed on labels. The author does, however, list calcium and phosphorus content of many common foods in the appendix, so this suggestion may not even be necessary.

LIFESTYLE AND EXERCISE Although not the crux of this plan, behavior is addressed as an important part of the osteoporosis prevention equation. The author promotes the theme of "taking control of your life." The book provides a self-evaluation questionnaire to determine whether you are drinking more than moderate amounts of alcohol, and it describes how much calcium loss drinking may be responsible for.

According to Mayes, behavior does not begin and end with the individual. She urges parents to set good examples to help children acquire good habits and avoid bad ones, so that the risk of osteoporosis will decrease for the next generation.

Exercise is advanced as a significant part of maintaining bone mass. Aerobic exercise accelerates blood flow to bones, increasing new bone growth. Weight-bearing exercises, which put beneficial stress on bones, also stimulate bone growth. Brisk walking fits both these categories and is touted as the best choice for many people. The author recommends medical approval before beginning a program of exercising three to four times per week, and she urges choosing an activity not only healthful but also enjoyable, one in which you can maintain interest.

WHY IT WORKS *Osteoporosis* is a quick A-to-Z guide for good bone building, a permanent reference guide, and a workable approach to maintaining strong bones throughout life. Most people will be able to implement most of the recommendations easily. Although the focus is on calcium and bone mass, the author's suggestions also fall within general health guidelines: strong bones are of little use if the rest of the body is ailing.

POTENTIAL DRAWBACKS   Probably the greatest deficit in this book is the lack of recipes or menu plans. While no diet should entirely take decision-making away from the dieter, the more specific the recommendations are, the better able the dieter is to make decisions.

The other suggestions are, for the most part, nutritionally sound but occasionally skate onto precarious ice. For example, the advice to use antacid tablets as a good calcium supplement, although tempered with warnings about some aluminum-containing antacids, is suspect because calcium needs an acid environment in order to be digested and absorbed by the body. Antacids are acid neutralizers and thus create the opposite kind of environment. The author also recommends eating ribs, which are a good calcium source but are also usually high in fat. Finally, she suggests that brown sugar is nutritionally more sound than white—when in fact the only difference between brown and white sugar is the inclusion of caramelizers in the former.

These problematic recommendations are aberrations in an otherwise scientifically sound work.

SECOND OPINIONS   "This is an excellent review of osteoporosis. The book covers the risk factors, the disease itself, and what people can do to prevent it. Food sources of calcium and calcium supplements are discussed, as is exercise, hormone treatment and other therapies. A chart of the calcium content of foods is included."

—Environmental Nutrition Newsletter

"*Osteoporosis* is a sound book on this physical disability for the average reader."

—ALA Booklist: The Professional
Multimedia Evaluation Service

THE CALCIUM CONNECTION
by Cedric Garland, M.D.,
Frank Garland, M.D., and
Ellen Thro
G. P. Putnam
New York: 1988

ABOUT THE AUTHORS Dr. Frank Garland is an assistant adjunct professor in community and family medicine at the University of California at San Diego and head of the occupational medicine department at San Diego's Naval Health Research Center. Dr. Cedric Garland is director of the epidemiology program of the Cancer Center at the University of California at San Diego, where he is an assistant professor. Ellen Thro is the author of two previous books.

OVERVIEW This book is the result of its authors' published research findings regarding the role of calcium and vitamin D in the prevention of certain kinds of cancer. Given the weight of this discovery, coupled with the fact that many people do not adequately absorb calcium simply because of the interaction of other foods they eat, the authors set out to create a plan for maximum calcium absorption through good food choices.

They offer a detailed analysis of the relationship between calcium and cancer. Calcium is a "means of cell communication" and prevents the kinds of cell division that can result in abnormal growths such as intestinal polyps. The authors explain that the connection between a high-fat diet and breast cancer is due to the fact that dietary fat blocks the absorption of calcium. They also describe calcium's role in regulating of blood pressure and preventing osteoporosis.

Next comes the crux of the book: a discussion of how calcium *consumed* does not necessarily translate to calcium *absorbed* and used. The authors identify those foods known to be "calcium robbers" and rank them by the average percentage of calcium each robs from the body. For example, the top three calcium robbers are bran, Swiss chard, and Brazil nuts.

On a positive note, they point out foods that help in the absorption and distribution of calcium throughout the body. Pectin,

170

for example, a substance found in many fruits and vegetables, attracts and delivers calcium to the large intestine and has been found to potentially reduce the risk of colon cancer.

To help the reader determine his or her particular calcium needs, the authors offer a series of profile questionnaires along with interpretational data. The interpretations consider eating habits in general, diet in particular, and environmental factors such as geographic location. Solar rays, for example, stimulate the skin to produce vitamin D, but overexposure can cause skin cancer.

With all of these individualized considerations in mind, *The Calcium Connection* then presents a diet plan ranging from as little as 1,200 calories per day (for those who want to lose weight) to 2,000 for women and 2,700 for men. The diet is high in calcium and vitamin D (which is necessary for calcium absorption) and low in foods that rob the body of those nutrients.

The recommended breakfast includes a calcium-rich breakfast shake, which begins a daily calcium intake of 800 milligrams. Though the authors suggest vitamin and mineral supplementation to ensure adequate overall nutrition, they insist that calcium and vitamin D should come from food sources to make certain that the body has the optimum absorption opportunity.

Because the authors encourage individuality, the diet plans are flexible. The charts of calcium-rich foods and calcium robbers make it easy to tailor your own eating plan. *The Calcium Connection* also discusses the importance of drinking enough water and getting water that is high in calcium.

NUTRITIONAL EVALUATION   An analysis of a two-day average on the 2,000-calorie plan showed calories a little low—1,865. These calories break down as follows:

```
Carbohydrates  . . . . . . . . . . . . . . . . . . . . . . . . . . . 61%
Protein . . . . . . . . . . . . . . . . . . . . . . . . . . . . . . . . . 17%
Fat  . . . . . . . . . . . . . . . . . . . . . . . . . . . . . . . . . . . 22%
Sodium  . . . . . . . . . . . . . . . . . . . . . . . . . . . . . 1,666 milligrams
Fiber  . . . . . . . . . . . . . . . . . . . . . . . . . . . . . . . . 15 grams
Cholesterol . . . . . . . . . . . . . . . . . . . . . . . . . . . 65 milligrams
```

All of the above fall within recommended goals except fiber, the result of the authors' recommendation to use white flour, a processed grain devoid of much of its fiber. Increasing whole grains and decreasing the use of processed flour should correct this

ANALYSIS OF 2-DAY MENU FOR FEMALE, AGE 35

The Calcium Connection

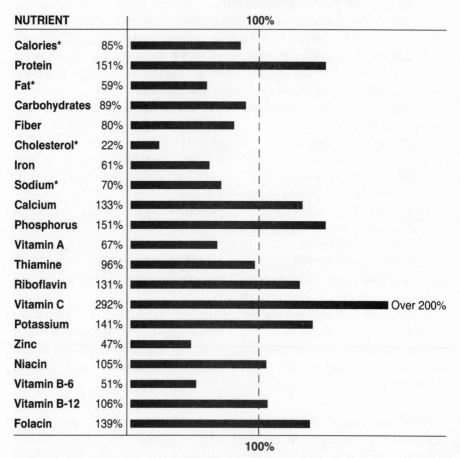

PERCENTAGE OF RA/RM

NUTRIENT		100%
Calories*	85%	
Protein	151%	
Fat*	59%	
Carbohydrates	89%	
Fiber	80%	
Cholesterol*	22%	
Iron	61%	
Sodium*	70%	
Calcium	133%	
Phosphorus	151%	
Vitamin A	67%	
Thiamine	96%	
Riboflavin	131%	
Vitamin C	292%	Over 200%
Potassium	141%	
Zinc	47%	
Niacin	105%	
Vitamin B-6	51%	
Vitamin B-12	106%	
Folacin	139%	

100%

*Recommended maximum allowance. Nutrient should not exceed 100%.

and would also help correct the diet's deficiencies in vitamin B-6, zinc, and iron. The only other nutrient this diet does not provide quite enough of is vitamin A; adding one carrot per day would make the necessary adjustment.

PRACTICALITY   The book is highly user friendly, its advice easy to understand and to follow. In addition to the lists of calcium robbers and calcium helpers, the appendix provides a listing of the calcium content of most foods (it even shows Evian as the bottled water highest in calcium). The meal plans offer variety and simplicity; the advice is to limit rather than totally eliminate most offending foods. Six ounces of wine, for example, are allowed per day.

LIFESTYLE AND EXERCISE   Though most of the book's emphasis is on *what* to do and not how to motivate yourself to do it, the authors do not ignore the fact that human beings are creatures of habit and that change is not always easy. The final chapter urges motivation and tries to inspire the reader to take the necessary action. It also emphasizes prevention and personal responsibility for self-care.

Like Maye's book, *The Calcium Connection* advises exercise that is both aerobic and weight-bearing. Exercise that increases circulation and puts beneficial stress on the backbone, pelvic bone, hip and leg bones helps promote calcium absorption into the bones.

WHY IT WORKS   *The Calcium Connection* takes a pragmatic approach to the problem of calcium and vitamin D absorption, distilling complex scientific data into a workable formula. The information is interesting, thorough, and useful. Calcium carbonate has been associated with the depletion of hydrochloric acid in the stomachs of people who do not have it in adequate amounts. This condition can also interefere with calcium absorption. The authors warn against *excessive* use of this calcium supplement.

The authors even list calcium information about fast food, frozen foods, and the drinking water of various major cities. They also caution against excessive exposure to the sun and against common environmental pollutants and other environmental hazards that increase the body's calcium needs, leaving less of the mineral for bone mass. Although the book is directed at an approach to a specific nutritional problem, it does not ignore other equally important health considerations. This diet, if adhered to, should promote health in a number of ways.

POTENTIAL DRAWBACKS   Most troubling is the statement that the absorbability of calcium carbonate "doesn't differ much from other calcium supplements." There is much evidence disputing this. Research at the University of Texas Health Science Center, for example, has demonstrated calcium citrate to have a higher solubility and thus a higher calcium availability than that of calcium carbonate. Furthermore, calcium carbonate has been associated with the depletion of hydrochloric acid in the stomach, which can interfere with calcium absorption. While the authors warn against excessive use of this calcium supplement, they do not go far enough.

The authors also recommend white rice over brown rice because white rice contains less of the calcium robber phytate. This, in my opinion, is not sound nutritional advice. Brown rice contains more niacin, calcium, phosphorous, magnesium, and fiber than white rice. I have a similar objection to their advising white flour over whole-wheat since readers following this book's dietary advice should be obtaining more than enough calcium to offset any losses from phytates or oxalic acid.

I was also disappointed that the recipes were not accompanied by a nutrient analysis; even a breakdown of calcium and vitamin D content would have been helpful.

SECOND OPINION   "The authors have accurately brought together all the critical facts about calcium in a complete program that can benefit everyone. Recommended."

—*Environment Nutrition Newsletter*

MEDICAL/HEALTH/SPECIALTY DIETS

CHEMOTHERAPY

A SUBSTANTIAL NUMBER OF DRUGS are used, sometimes along with radiation, in the treatment of cancer. While they have the potential for causing remission of the disease, these medicines frequently produce unpleasant side effects—most commonly loss of appetite, nausea and vomiting, diarrhea, constipation, dehydration, and difficulty chewing or swallowing. All of these symptoms can interfere with proper diet; poor nutrition in turn will impair both the effectiveness of the medical treatment and the body's ability to defend against drug side effects.

Additionally, both the disease and its treatment may cause changes in the body's ability to ingest and utilize food, in part because of psychological and physiological stresses. In most cases, the patient's energy and nutrient needs are greater than normal, and thus more calories are required.

Patients are not always as aware as they should be about the importance of nutrition. The following book should help.

NUTRITION FOR THE CHEMOTHERAPY PATIENT

Ernest H. Rosenbaum, M.D. and
Janet L. Ramstack, Ph.D.
Bull Publishing Company
Palo Alto, California: 1990

ABOUT THE AUTHORS   Dr. Rosenbaum is associate chief of medicine at Mount Zion Hospital and Medical Center and director of oncology at French Hospital, both in San Francisco. He is medical director of the San Francisco Regional Center Foundation and a clinical professor of medicine at the University of California, San Francisco. His other books include *A Comprehensive Guide for Cancer Patients and their Families, Living with Cancer,* and *Can You Prevent Cancer?*

Dr. Ramstack received her doctorate in public health from Tulane University. A registered dietitian, she has most recently been assistant professor and director of food service and dietetics programs for Morehead State University in Kentucky. She is a lecturer on nutrition and cancer and has appeared on radio and television. She conceived this book from her experiences helping her husband overcome Hodgkin's disease and the complications of chemotherapy.

OVERVIEW   The goal of this book is to enable the chemotherapy patient to eat in a manner that promotes optimum nutrition and maximum drug effectiveness, working toward the ultimate goal of remission and healing. Rosenbaum and Ramstack provide general eating guidelines for chemotherapy patients, specific dietary advice for dealing with various side effects, and comprehensive descriptions of more than 40 chemotherapy drugs.

The authors recommend that cancer patients eat a diet composed of 50 to 60 percent complex carbohydrates, 15 to 20 percent protein, and 20 to 30 percent fat, although the stress of chemotherapy may increase protein needs. Chemotherapy patients also commonly require more than the RDA of specific vitamins, but they must be cautious in using vitamin and mineral supplements to avoid potential toxicity and adverse drug-nutrient reactions. According to the authors, patients can get adequate nutrition without these risks by eating a wide variety of nutrient-dense foods (those with a high concentration of nutrients per calorie).

Rosenbaum and Ramstack provide a simple "swallowing training program" for chemotherapy patients with swallowing difficulties, to enable them to consume sufficient calories and nutrients. They offer 25 recipes to accommodate swallowing difficulties, along with 17 recipes for cooking with commercial food supplements. In all, the book includes 168 recipes, among them American and ethnic, meat and meatless main dishes, salads, soups, sauces, dairy and egg dishes, muffins, quick breads, and beverages. Total calories and protein are listed for each. To ensure that patients get the necessary levels of protein and total calories, the authors encourage desserts for lunch as well as dinner and snacks between meals and at bedtime.

Besides impaired swallowing, the authors discuss other problems common to chemotherapy patients that can cause nutritional deficiencies: loss of appetite, nausea and vomiting, taste changes, sore or ulcerated mouth or throat, chewing difficulty, kidney stones, glucose intolerance, lactose intolerance, gluten intolerance, diarrhea, constipation, bleeding and ulcers in the gastrointestinal tract, steatorrhea (fat in the stool), and dehydration. They offer tips for alleviating such problems, including customized eating plans that match the patient's caloric and nutrient requirements and food tolerances. Some examples:

- A *lactose-free diet* for chemotherapy patients who develop intolerance to milk products.

- A *gluten restricted diet* for those who develop a sensitivity to wheat products.

- A *long-chain-triglyceride restricted fat diet* to reduce the malabsorption of fat and relieve symptoms of steatorrhea.

- A *cholesterol/fat restricted diet* for patients who must lower their serum cholesterol.

- A *kidney-stone prevention diet* for the many chemotherapy patients who develop this painful condition.

• *A soft food/pureed food diet* for those with chewing and swallowing problems.

To help the reader understand the changes in his or her body and learn what to do about them, the authors also provide insight as to how drug side effects are monitored.

NUTRITIONAL EVALUATION   The book has neither menus nor formal dietary programs. The eating guidelines, however, are excellent and the foods they emphasize should promote a nutritionally sound diet.

PRACTICALITY   The book contains helpful, easily understood charts. It can be used in conjunction with a registered dietitian or to assist a doctor, primary caregiver, or the patient in making food choices that can be tolerated and that will defend against nutritional inadequacies.

LIFESTYLE AND EXERCISE   The book is written in an optimistic and encouraging tone to put the reader in a positive frame of mind. It offers insight and advice that the cancer patient can implement in order to make a difference in his or her own life.

Exercise is often not possible for chemotherapy patients; it does not become a priority until after recovery. For this reason, it is not discussed.

WHY IT WORKS   The tips for cooking and for label reading are clear and useful, and the extensiveness of the various dietary modifications makes this an excellent workbook for patient, caregiver, or physician. It contains a wealth of information that would be impossible for any doctor to convey to a patient during the time limitations of office visits.

With anything as frightening and often mystifying as cancer and chemotherapy, patient awareness and involvement can make a profound difference in terms of the potential for recovery and overall quality of life. Chemotherapy patients need to feel a commitment to their own treatment; the detailed dietary information in this book gives them the assurance that they *can* make a difference.

POTENTIAL DRAWBACKS   I found no significant drawbacks in this work.

SECOND OPINION   *"Nutrition for the Chemotherapy Patient* is essential for every cancer patient on chemotherapy. It is the only source available of this vital information on the nutrition effects of chemotherapeutic agents."

—*Fredrick F. Mayer, R.Ph., M.P.H.*
President, Pharmacists Planning Services Inc.
Past President, California Public Health Association

MEDICAL/HEALTH/SPECIALTY DIETS

CHOLESTEROL REDUCTION

CORONARY HEART DISEASE is the leading cause of death in the United States today, and high cholesterol is one of its most significant risk factors; more than half of the U.S. adult population, in fact, is at increased risk of heart attack because of high cholesterol. A blood cholesterol level of more than 240 milligrams per deciliter of blood can more than *double* your risk of coronary heart disease.

Most Americans are aware that high cholesterol is a health hazard, but they do not necessarily know exactly what cholesterol is or how it can be controlled. Cholesterol is a waxy, odorless substance found in animal food sources, most prominently beef, poultry, and dairy products, and also produced within your own body. Cholesterol is a necessary substance in the body, essential to the formation of brain tissue, nerve tissue, cell membranes, and hormones. But when consumed in excess through food sources, cholesterol can have a damaging effect on blood vessels.

Cholesterol is transported through the bloodstream by two different kinds of lipoproteins (fat-carrying protein molecules): high-density lipoproteins (HDL) and low-density lipoproteins (LDL). HDL carries cholesterol back to the liver, which uses it for key body functions. LDL tends to carry some of the cholesterol into the walls of the arteries, where it can accumulate with other fatty substances, forming yellowish plaque that can narrow the size of the opening through which blood flows. Over time these deposits can totally obstruct the flow of blood. Such obstructions can occur in any artery anywhere in the body, with serious consequences, such as hypertension and stroke. Coronary arteries are particularly vulnerable to such blockage, and the consequence is extremely serious: heart attack.

High cholesterol and plaque build-up cause no symptoms at first, but gradually, as the heart muscle is increasingly deprived of oxygen and nutrients, a common symptom is chest pain (known medically as angina pectoris).

Even if severe blockage occurs before the symptoms alert you, it may not be too late to stop—and even to reverse—the damage. It is therefore not surprising that a great deal has been written about how to reduce serum cholesterol. From this body of literature I have selected three books that have helped many people begin to control their cholesterol.

CONTROLLING CHOLESTEROL

by Kenneth H. Cooper, M.D., M.P.H.
Bantam Books
New York: 1988

ABOUT THE AUTHOR   Dr. Cooper received his medical degree from the University of Oklahoma School of Medicine and his master's in public health from Harvard University. He has written numerous books about aerobic exercise, including *Aerobics*, the landmark book that coined the term. He is founder of the Cooper Clinic and director of the Aerobics Center in Dallas. His aerobics system is used by the U.S. Navy and Air Force.

OVERVIEW   Cooper's stated objective in this book is to help people learn the latest and most important information and techniques available to help fight elevated blood cholesterol, which he refers to as "killer cholesterol." He tells the reader that the key to good health is prevention; specifically, that lowering cholesterol before it becomes life-threatening is the best medicine of all. Even if you already have atherosclerosis (fatty deposits in the arteries), Cooper points out that it can be stopped and even reversed through the right lifestyle changes.

The book provides a simplified description of the basic facts about cholesterol: what it is, how it is produced, how good and bad cholesterol differ and how to distinguish between them, and how diet and exercise affect total blood cholesterol. This includes a discussion about the importance of a low cholesterol ratio: total cholesterol (which should be as low as possible) to HDL "good" cholesterol (which should be as high as possible). The lower the cholesterol ratio, the better. For example, someone with total cholesterol of 200 and an HDL of 50 has a ratio of 4.0; someone with total cholesterol of 180 and an HDL of 60 has a healthier ratio of 3.0.

Cooper also covers the significance of triglycerides and provides a question-and-answer section about the best ways to test blood cholesterol, as well as tests to assess your knowledge of cholesterol and nutrition. Cooper advises talking to your physician about achieving the right cholesterol balance.

In discussing the role of age and heredity in cholesterol and heart disease, Cooper stresses that the most influential factors for most people are the controllable ones: diet and lifestyle. He recognizes the need for cholesterol-lowering drugs in some cases, but maintains—citing scientific studies—that for most people a change in diet and lifestyle is not only the safer method of controlling cholesterol, but even the more effective method. He prioritizes the attack on high cholesterol in this manner:

1. Eat a low-cholesterol diet.

2. Reduce total body-fat percentage through weight reduction and aerobic exercise, and thus reduce the fat in the blood.

3. If necessary, take cholesterol-lowering drugs, niacin, or other supplements under a doctor's supervision.

With nutrition as the most significant factor in determining total cholesterol for most people, Cooper provides extensive dietary advice. He offers three levels of fat and cholesterol restrictions.

The Basic Diet is for the average person who wants to maintain or achieve healthful cholesterol and blood lipid (fat) levels; fat accounts for 20–30 percent of total calories (a level within RDA guidelines). This diet contains 300 milligrams of cholesterol per day.

The Moderate Diet is for people who, after eight weeks on the Basic Diet, find themselves unable to achieve an adequate cholesterol reduction (Cooper considers this to be anything less than a 10 percent cholesterol reduction after eight weeks). This diet reduces fat to 15–20 percent and lowers cholesterol intake to 200 milligrams per day.

The Strict Diet is for those unable to adequately control cholesterol on either of the previous diets. Here, fat accounts for only 10–15 percent of total daily calories, and cholesterol is down to 100 milligrams.

All three diets are variations of the same theme: high complex carbohydrates, healthy amounts of oat products (including oat bran), and an emphasis on monounsaturated fats, which have been found to lower total cholesterol. He provides specific menus with categorized food lists for easy substitutions. For example, a small amount of peanut butter can replace a serving of tuna.

These extensive menus are accompanied by 82 low-fat recipes, including quick chicken and fish entrees, other main dishes, soups, vegetable dishes, salad dressings, breakfast items, sauces, baked goods, and desserts. Each recipe contains information about calories, fat, cholesterol, and food exchange. Cooper also furnishes general advice on low-fat cooking and general guidelines for cutting dietary fat within each food group.

These three diets are not only designed to lower cholesterol consumption but also to lower total dietary fat, thus reducing body fat and blood lipids, the program's second cholesterol-reducing tool.

Cooper also details the major factors besides dietary fat that raise or lower cholesterol. He tells us that coffee, in addition to its other health hazards, has been found to raise LDL "bad" cholesterol and that smoking can lower HDL "good" cholesterol. On the other hand, a moderate amount of alcohol (two ounces per day) has been found to *raise* HDL cholesterol—though Cooper tempers these findings with the potential health dangers of alcohol and reminds the reader that aerobic exercise accomplishes the same positive goal without the negative side effects. Finally, emotional stress has been found to raise total blood cholesterol, according to studies Cooper cites. With that in mind, Cooper presents stress antidotes, including regular aerobic exercise and relaxation techniques.

If these menu plans and other lifestyle modifications fail to reduce cholesterol sufficiently, he suggests talking to your physician about implementing a more aggressive cholesterol-controlling plan, including the possible use of niacin and cholesterol-reducing drugs. Cooper stresses the importance of understanding the principles behind drug therapy and of learning as much as you can about the available treatments so that you can be an active rather than a passive patient. This begins with insisting upon a second blood cholesterol test to make absolutely certain that cholesterol levels are not responding to dietary modifications. Being an active patient also means monitoring your own body whenever you have to use any drug and knowing as much about the medication as possible. Cooper discusses the latest cholesterol-lowering drugs, how they work, their potential side effects, and the drug combinations that have been found to be effective.

This book contains a wealth of information about cholesterol and heart disease, including insights about the connection between cholesterol and cancer and the latest advice about children and cholesterol—when to start serum cholesterol testing of your child, how to interpret the results along with your pediatrician, and how to modify your child's diet if cholesterol is too high.

Throughout the book, Cooper uses interesting case histories to illustrate his points, yet he presents both sides of every issue before giving recommendations.

NUTRITIONAL EVALUATION   An analysis of a two-day average found the calories within an acceptable range but slightly higher than the author's recommendations. Those calories break down as follows:

Carbohydrates	51%
Protein	25%
Fat	24%
Sodium	3,328 milligrams
Fiber	37 grams
Cholesterol	408 milligrams

Protein is high and carbohydrates are low by current standards, but both meet the pre-1989 goals that were in effect when the book was written. Fat is well within acceptable guidelines, but cholesterol, surprisingly, is high (the inclusion of shrimp on one of the menus probably accounts for much of that). Sodium is also well above recommended goals. On the plus side, fiber is well above the recommended range. This diet meets 100 percent of the RDA for all important vitamins and minerals except for zinc, which is still above two-thirds of the RDA.

PRACTICALITY   This book is easy to read and well organized, with step-by-step procedures and advice for lowering total blood cholesterol. The menus are simple and easy to follow, as are the corresponding recipes.

Cooper does not directly address the issues of restaurant meals

ANALYSIS OF 2-DAY MENU FOR MALE, AGE 35

Controlling Cholesterol

PERCENTAGE OF RA/RM

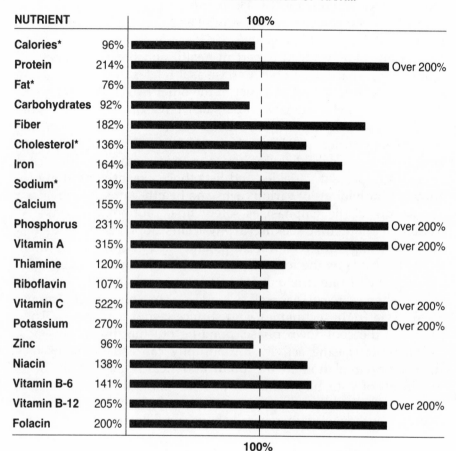

NUTRIENT		
Calories*	96%	
Protein	214%	Over 200%
Fat*	76%	
Carbohydrates	92%	
Fiber	182%	
Cholesterol*	136%	
Iron	164%	
Sodium*	139%	
Calcium	155%	
Phosphorus	231%	Over 200%
Vitamin A	315%	Over 200%
Thiamine	120%	
Riboflavin	107%	
Vitamin C	522%	Over 200%
Potassium	270%	Over 200%
Zinc	96%	
Niacin	138%	
Vitamin B-6	141%	
Vitamin B-12	205%	Over 200%
Folacin	200%	

100%

*Recommended maximum allowance. Nutrient should not exceed 100%.

or eating when traveling, but the diet itself allows for flexibility. Once familiar with the guidelines, you should be able to eat out or on the road without compromising your cholesterol.

The advice in this book is sound and reasonable, and the entire family can follow the diet program, enjoying health benefits whether or not they need to lower their cholesterol.

LIFESTYLE AND EXERCISE   Cooper provides relaxation tips to reduce cholesterol-elevating emotional stress and case histories to lend encouragement and insights for fine-tuning your lifestyle and taking charge of your health. He points to knowledge as the base from which you can control cholesterol and prevent heart disease—and then delivers that knowledge.

As an acknowledged expert in health and fitness, Cooper devotes a lot of space to aerobic exercise as it relates to cholesterol and heart disease (more so than either of the other two cholesterol books in this section). He begins with persuasive reasons to exercise—the specifics of how it elevates HDL good cholesterol, lowers triglycerides, burns calories—then recommends 20 to 30 minutes three to four times per week, detailing those exercises most beneficial. He discusses important variables and lists those exercises most appropriate for individuals of various ages and health status.

Above all, he emphasizes safety first, cautioning against exercising without first seeking a physician's approval. Cooper discusses the importance of warm-ups and explains how to do them safely. He explains the formula for calculating a safe and appropriate target heart rate (the maximum rate you want to get your heart to beat when exercising) as well as his 4 S's—stretching, shoes (proper ones), style (right technique), and surface (avoid hard ones). Then he covers the cool-down phase, pointing out that this is the most critical time: ceasing activity too abruptly can cause dangerously inadequate circulation to the brain and heart, since as much as 60 percent of your blood may be pooled below the waist. He adds warnings about using a sauna or steam room immediately after a vigorous workout and, in general, about overdoing exercise.

WHY IT WORKS   Cooper helps the reader assess his or her heart disease risks and then outlines ways to measurably reduce them. This comprehensive study of cholesterol and heart disease takes complex scientific data and distills them into an understandable and educational narrative, using clever and vivid metaphors—for example, the liver is a shipbuilder, the supply ship is very-low-density lipoprotein (VLDL), which carries triglyceride cargo to the cells for energy needs and later becomes LDL (bad cholesterol) when present in excess amounts in the bloodstream.

This book is a complete approach to a healthy cardiovascular system, stressing a reduction in convenience foods and a greater reliance on natural whole grains; vegetables (steamed for maximum nutrients and taste); fruits (whole fruits rather than juices from which much of the fiber has been depleted); monounsaturated oils; and fresh fish, which contain cholesterol-lowering omega-3 fish oil.

The diet itself with its built-in modifications is designed to get results, and so is Cooper's philosophy. He tells the reader that cholesterol *can* be controlled with proper diet, exercise, and a working knowledge and understanding of cholesterol, blood fats, and their impact on cardiovascular health.

POTENTIAL DRAWBACKS   The only drawback is that the Strict Diet plan may be deficient in some essential nutrients, especially calcium, perhaps requiring the dieter to use vitamin and mineral supplementation.

SECOND OPINIONS   "The book contains accurate information in an easily readable style. It also provides tools for patients' follow-up: menus, recipes, and food composition tables. This book can be recommended for patients with elevated blood cholesterol levels."

—*Nutrition and the M.D.*

"*Controlling Cholesterol* belongs on the bookshelf of every home and office in America. If the recommendations of this book could be understood and practiced by each and every American, the epidemic of cardiovascular disease we are presently experiencing might end up being a footnote in medical history."

—*Current Diet Review*

"Despite minor drawbacks, *Controlling Cholesterol* achieves its goal—to provide readers with the knowledge to take control of their health. The book is an informative and excellent resource for educated and concerned consumers as well as health professionals. Knowledge certainly is power. Recommended."

—*Environmental Nutrition Newsletter*

COUNT OUT CHOLESTEROL

by Art Ulene, M.D.
Feeling Fine Programs, Inc.
Los Angeles: 1989

ABOUT THE AUTHOR   Dr. Art Ulene is a graduate of the UCLA School of Medicine. He is best known for his medical segments on NBC TV's *Today Show* and for his syndicated medical reports, "Feeling Fine," which are featured on newscasts in more than 100 cities. He is spokesperson for the American Medical Association's Campaign Against Cholesterol. His book is the official AMA book on the subject of cholesterol management.

OVERVIEW   This book sets out to provide a means for most people with high cholesterol to significantly reduce their cholesterol within 30 days. Ulene believes that there is no single way to lower cholesterol for everyone—that different people develop high cholesterol for different reasons—but that most people can control cholesterol without the use of drugs by modifying their diet with a substantial reduction in saturated fat and an increase in soluble fiber.

He presents cross-cultural data to illustrate cholesterol risks and provides some insight into the cholesterol numbers game. The risk of a heart attack, according to the author, begins to rise as the cholesterol level reaches about 150 and increases dramatically once it exceeds 200. On the other hand, for every 1 percent *reduction* in the cholesterol level, the chances of a heart attack decrease by 2 percent.

With this incentive in place, Ulene discusses what cholesterol is and some reasons why its level may rise too high in the blood. Citing various research studies, including those from the Multiple Risk Factor Intervention Trial and the Lipid Research Clinic, he describes the factors that determine cholesterol level, beginning with the amount of total dietary fat—especially saturated fat—along with dietary fiber and the amount of cholesterol manufactured in the liver. Although he points out that such uncontrollable factors as heredity, sex, and age also have influence, the emphasis is on those elements over which the individual has control. This includes elevating HDL (good) cholesterol as well as lowering LDL (bad) cholesterol. HDL cholesterol, which in high levels lowers the risk of heart disease, is suppressed by smoking and being overweight; thus many people can elevate their HDL level by reducing to an ideal weight and quitting smoking. Exercise, according to the author, has also been found to elevate HDL cholesterol.

Ulene uses the National Cholesterol Education Program guidelines in making recommendations about goals for lowering LDL and total cholesterol. He helps demystify cholesterol numbers by providing a formula for calculating the total cholesterol/HDL ratio, with the goal of making that ratio as small as possible. The author recommends having your blood cholesterol tested so that you know where you stand; he gives some advice about which tests are the most accurate and the most cost effective.

The cholesterol-lowering diet itself is presented in the form of charts, based upon the concept of a maximum number of grams of saturated fat in the diet each day in order to lower cholesterol. He refers to this saturated fat limit as SF1 and tells the reader how to calculate the limit based upon height, weight, sex, and activity level. Food lists provide choices based upon fat content in relation to SF1.

Ulene discusses food groups that are particularly troublesome for those trying to lower cholesterol. He gives advice on controlling amounts for those who prefer not to entirely give up such foods as beef, seafood, milk, cheese, and ice cream.

The other major goal of this diet is to ensure adequate daily intake of soluble fiber. Ulene calls this daily fiber minimum the SF2 and shows the reader how to determine SF2 and how to get that soluble fiber. He discusses the pros and cons of fiber supplements as a secondary source.

Ulene provides seven recipes using foods on his SF1 and SF2 food lists, offers advice on reading food labels to find hidden sources of saturated fat, and gives tips on dining out while adhering to the cholesterol-lowering program.

The book contains a 30-day diary to help you monitor your progress. If you experience no progress, Ulene suggests reducing your SF1 from 10 percent of total calories to 7 percent.

The diary can also help your physician determine how responsive your body is to the lowered dietary cholesterol approach; though changes in eating habits work for the vast majority of people, they do not work for everyone. Since physicians often prescribe cholesterol-lowering drugs to those patients who do not respond to dietary modifications, the author details those drugs: how they work, how they differ, and their potential side effects.

These drugs are presented only as a last resort. Diet and other lifestyle changes are the focus of Ulene's program. In addition to dietary changes, he suggests cholesterol-lowering measures involving nonsmoking, alcohol moderation, and regular exercise.

NUTRITIONAL EVALUATION   An analysis of a sample day's menu found the calories within an acceptable range, broken down as follows:

```
Carbohydrates ............................ 49%
Protein .................................... 29%
Fat ........................................ 22%
Sodium ................................... 1,916 milligrams
Fiber ..................................... 30 grams
Cholesterol ............................... 330 milligrams
```

Protein is rather high and carbohydrates are too low, even based on the pre-1989 goals in effect when this book was published. Fat is well within acceptable goals, but cholesterol, surprisingly, is higher— about 10 percent above the recognized upper limit. I would suggest modifying the diet by halving the protein portions and doubling vegetable serving sizes. Fiber and sodium are both within acceptable goals. All important vitamins and minerals meet 100 percent of the RDA.

PRACTICALITY   There are no rigid menus or special recipes to prepare. The general diet principles of low saturated fat and high soluble fiber are flexible and should be accessible to most people. There are no foods you have to completely avoid. Ulene, in fact, makes the point that an occasional deviation from the diet won't raise total blood cholesterol significantly.

The necessity of keeping notes on food intake, though helpful and desirable, may be tedious for some.

LIFESTYLE AND EXERCISE   For those who do not find recording their daily food intake tedious, this practice can be an effective behavioral modification tool, especially since the diary included in the book contains specific advice about eating and lifestyle changes in order to lower cholesterol.

Ulene urges the reader to take control, to make a commitment to reduce the risk of heart disease; then he provides sample menus that illustrate exactly how to do so. For anyone with the motivation,

ANALYSIS OF 1-DAY MENU FOR MALE, AGE 35

Count Out Cholesterol

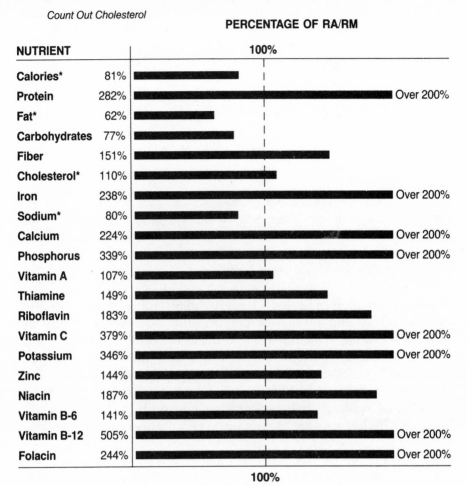

PERCENTAGE OF RA/RM

NUTRIENT			100%	
Calories*	81%			
Protein	282%			Over 200%
Fat*	62%			
Carbohydrates	77%			
Fiber	151%			
Cholesterol*	110%			
Iron	238%			Over 200%
Sodium*	80%			
Calcium	224%			Over 200%
Phosphorus	339%			Over 200%
Vitamin A	107%			
Thiamine	149%			
Riboflavin	183%			
Vitamin C	379%			Over 200%
Potassium	346%			Over 200%
Zinc	144%			
Niacin	187%			
Vitamin B-6	141%			
Vitamin B-12	505%			Over 200%
Folacin	244%			Over 200%

100%

*Recommended maximum allowance. Nutrient should not exceed 100%.

this is perhaps the best kind of behavioral modification: to be shown a simple and comprehensive method.

The author recommends a moderate amount of aerobic activity, such as brisk walking, bicycling, and swimming. He advises rotating exercises and picking those you enjoy. He leaves the specifics to your physician, whom he suggests you consult before beginning an exercise program.

WHY IT WORKS Reducing saturated fat and increasing fiber is good nutritional advice for all Americans—not only for lowering cholesterol but for promoting overall good health. The high-complex-carbohydrate diet will also promote weight loss and weight control, which in turn helps reduce cholesterol. This is not a quick-fix approach, relying on some magic food such as oat bran to single-handedly reduce cholesterol. It is a plan designed to become a permanent part of your lifestyle.

The book is easy to read and well organized. The charts are useful and the directions on how to use them are clear. Finally, the discussion of cholesterol-reducing drugs is excellent; since many doctors do prescribe them, a working knowledge of their effects and side effects can be valuable.

POTENTIAL DRAWBACKS Considering the importance of exercise in elevating HDL cholesterol and in weight control—an important part of controlling total cholesterol—this book would have benefited from a more comprehensive section about exercise. Also, more recipes would have been helpful.

Additionally, I found an omission and an error in Ulene's nutritional information. His list of high-cholesterol seafood does not include squid, and his list of polyunsaturated oils incorrectly includes canola oil, which is a monounsaturated fat. Finally, there is no discussion of monounsaturated fats and their ability to help lower total cholesterol. This omission may be due to the fact that this book reflects the AMA view, which requires extraordinary amounts of research before accepting any finding. Otherwise the book gets high marks for accuracy and comprehensiveness.

SECOND OPINION *"Count Out Cholesterol* is highly recommended for readers who want to lower their serum cholesterol levels. Readers should be cautioned to watch their total fat intake as well as their saturated fat intake, but, overall, the recommendations in this book will help most people reduce their risk of heart disease."

—Current Diet Review

THE 8-WEEK CHOLESTEROL CURE

by Robert E. Kowalski
Harper & Row Publishers
New York: 1987

ABOUT THE AUTHOR   A medical writer for more than 20 years, Kowalski has written educational materials used in hospitals and clinics. His two other books are *Cholesterol and Children* and *The 8-Week Cholesterol Cook Book.*

This book is the result of Kowalski's own bout with high cholesterol, which led to a heart attack and two coronary bypass surgeries by the time he was 41. According to Kowalski, he developed a program that enabled him to lower his cholesterol from 284 to 169, cutting his heart attack risk in half.

OVERVIEW   *The 8-Week Cholesterol Cure* begins with a discussion of the relationship between diet and coronary heart disease along with a definition of HDL and LDL cholesterol and triglyceride levels. Then Kowalski presents his three-pronged approach to lowering cholesterol: low-fat diet, increased dietary fiber, and vitamin therapy.

His low-fat dietary recommendations are to limit meat servings to four ounces a day and restrict milk to low-fat or nonfat varieties in order to cut fat intake to 20 percent of total calories, and cholesterol to no more than 250 milligrams per day (both well within the RDA). He suggests eating as much fruit, vegetables, and pasta as you can without gaining weight, and gives some general tips on weight control, such as always sitting while eating and using a smaller-sized plate to make meals look bigger. Kowalski offers 91 recipes, including muffins, breads, meat and seafood entrees, turkey dishes, fruit milkshakes, breakfasts, and desserts, along with food charts and label-reading lessons to ensure that the reader can pinpoint saturated fat on the dietary landscape.

The fiber aspect of Kowalski's program begins by differentiating water-soluble fiber from insoluble and describing the role of dietary fiber in controlling cholesterol. Kowalski recommends eating three high-fiber oat-bran muffins per day, and he supplies 12 different muffin recipes using low-fat milk and egg substitutes. He also lists other foods and food products that contain high soluble fiber and discusses nonfood sources of soluble fiber, such as guar gum and Metamucil.

The vitamin therapy component of the 8-Week Cholesterol Cure focuses on niacin and its role in lowering cholesterol. According to research Kowalski cites, niacin not only lowers LDL and VLDL (both harmful cholesterol) but also lowers harmful triglycerides and raises good HDL cholesterol. Using a table for illustration, Kowalski describes how to take niacin for cholesterol control, starting out with small dosages and gradually increasing to as much as 3,000 milligrams per day. Since there are potential side effects from such large doses, the author suggests consulting a physician and having a liver function test performed after two months of taking the vitamin supplement. He also recommends a time-release form of niacin, that provides better results with fewer side effects.

Kowalski also discusses the role stress plays in cholesterol and offers techniques for reducing negative stress.

According to Kowalski, those who adhere to this program can enjoy the following rewards: weight control without deprivation, a cholesterol level that will drop at least 20 percent and as much as 40 percent, and improved chances for a long life.

NUTRITIONAL EVALUATION The author does not include specific menus—he believes that no one pays attention to such menus. He does, however, show several days of what he considers typical food intake on his diet, demonstrating the wide variety of foods you can eat while staying within his recommended guidelines. I have analyzed two such days, using standard portion sizes where none were specified. Thus, the results are, at best, an estimate. The 1,547 calories appear to be an acceptable range for the author's specific body requirements. A larger man would need more. The breakdown is as follows:

Carbohydrates	56%
Protein	24%
Fat	20%
Sodium	2,740 milligrams
Fiber	64 grams
Cholesterol	172 milligrams

ANALYSIS OF 1-DAY MENU FOR MALE, AGE 45

The 8-Week Cholesterol Cure

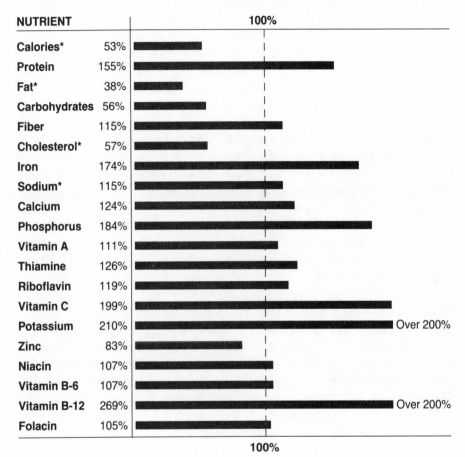

NUTRIENT	PERCENTAGE OF RA/RM
Calories*	53%
Protein	155%
Fat*	38%
Carbohydrates	56%
Fiber	115%
Cholesterol*	57%
Iron	174%
Sodium*	115%
Calcium	124%
Phosphorus	184%
Vitamin A	111%
Thiamine	126%
Riboflavin	119%
Vitamin C	199%
Potassium	210% (Over 200%)
Zinc	83%
Niacin	107%
Vitamin B-6	107%
Vitamin B-12	269% (Over 200%)
Folacin	105%

*Recommended maximum allowance. Nutrient should not exceed 100%.

Fat, cholesterol, carbohydrates, and fiber all meet established health goals. Protein is slightly high, but acceptable because of the high carbohydrate and low fat levels. Sodium, however, is too high—because of portions of cured ham and tomato juice (foods that would probably not be an everyday choice).

All important micronutrients meet 100 percent of the RDA except for zinc, which is above two-thirds of the RDA.

PRACTICALITY The book is easy to read, with a clear and easy-to-follow format. The program itself should be a reasonable and accessible approach for most people. The suggestions for reducing saturated fats are reasonable and should be effective. High-fat treats such as ice cream are allowed, provided the dieter balances them against total daily cholesterol intake, and the simplicity of getting 50 grams per day of soluble fiber in the form of muffins is a convenience for busy people. These muffins are relatively easy to make and to pack for work or travel; they last several days without refrigeration and can survive in a motel room in a plastic bag on ice. The author also makes a helpful suggestion about using Metamucil as a handy way of ensuring adequate daily fiber while traveling.

Kowalski uses a developmental approach: starting with current eating habits and modifying them where necessary, rather than starting from square one. He offers a number of suggestions for grocery shopping, restaurant eating (including ethnic cuisines), and accommodating your dietary needs at dinner parties.

On the down side, the recipes lack nutritional analyses, and some do not include serving-size information, making it difficult to calculate daily fat intake.

LIFESTYLE AND EXERCISE Kowalski advocates the power of positive thinking. "Look for the good in everything," he writes. "Turn those lemons into lemonade." He backs up this advice with illustrations of common negative thoughts about diet and life along with constructive positive alternative ways to look at the situation. He recommends positive imaging techniques for ideal body weight and cholesterol levels, along with a food diary to help monitor eating patterns and achieve those goals.

The behavioral aspects of this program do not end there. Since stress can have a direct effect on arterial health and heart disease risk, Kowalski offers strategies for reducing the number and intensity of stressful incidents, and finding ways to relax.

The book ends with a motivational pitch for making the recommended changes in your life, understanding that they could be life-saving. The author asks if doughnuts and Béarnaise sauce are worth a year—or even a month, week, or day—of your life.

Kowalski also recognizes the role that exercise can play in raising good HDL cholesterol and in improving general health and reducing the heart attack risk. He recommends regular exercise three to five times per week, with a physician's approval, but leaves it up to the reader to figure out what to do and how to do it.

WHY IT WORKS   This book is easy to follow, with clear and effective food charts. Kowalski presents scientifically researched information and cites his sources. His program is one of moderation and reasonableness. He recommends enjoying such treats as shellfish, low-fat frozen yogurt, and alcoholic beverages in moderation rather than trying to eliminate them completely.

Following his program can reduce your consumption of saturated fat, which should reduce total cholesterol. The use of niacin can help lower the amount of cholesterol produced in the liver. Unlike many other diet books, Kowalski *does* distinguish between polyunsaturated and monounsaturated oils and recommends the latter, which have been shown to help maintain good HDL cholesterol levels.

The author's nutritional advice should also promote overall good health. He pays careful attention to calcium and iron needs, keeps added salt and large amounts of sugar out of his recipes, and urges eight glasses of water per day.

POTENTIAL DRAWBACKS   Alcoholics, people with gout, colitis, or abnormal heart rhythm, or anyone else at risk for liver disease should not consider taking niacin. Everyone else should do so *only under the close supervision of a doctor*, since large doses can produce druglike effects. (*The Annals of Internal Medicine* recently reported a case in which a man, in trying to control cholesterol, switched from regular niacin to long-acting niacin and within three days suffered jaundice and liver failure. This, of course, may very well be an isolated case.) Kowalski does recommend medical supervision but then proceeds to tell the reader exactly how to self-prescribe niacin, a seeming contradiction.

Another contradiction: at one point Kowalski claims that carrots have no effect on blood fats. Later he cites a study by U.S. Department of Agriculture scientists that concluded that "carrot pectin" lowered cholesterol levels.

His list of monounsaturated fats is incomplete, leaving out canola oil. Another omission is leaving squid off a list of high-cholesterol seafoods. Another misleading statement about seafood is the recommendation to use imitation crab. While low in fat and cholesterol, imitation crab is often high in sodium and nutritionally inferior to the food it replaces.

Although most of Kowalski's suggestions are in the spirit of moderation and pragmatism, his directive to completely avoid cheese is extreme and may be impractical. There are a number of fat-free and low-fat cheeses that, in moderation, should not obstruct your efforts to control cholesterol.

Finally, this book leaves a lot up to the dieter. The author tells you to create your own menus from the recipes and other information in the book. While this may help independent-minded people who don't appreciate a lot of imposed structure, it may work against others who need more specific direction.

SECOND OPINION "This is a valuable tool for people with elevated cholesterol levels, as long as readers do not take niacin on their own. Side effects must be monitored carefully by a physician. With that in mind, heart patients as well as their doctors may find the book instructive. Borderline recommended."

—*Environmental Nutrition Newsletter*

MEDICAL/HEALTH/SPECIALTY DIETS

DIABETES

ONE OF THE THREE MOST serious diseases in America (along with heart disease and cancer), diabetes is, unfortunately, a disease on the rise. In the last 45 years, the number of cases has increased tenfold. Every year about six million new cases of diabetes are diagnosed, along with an estimated five million Americans who don't know they have it.

Diabetes is characterized by abnormally high blood-sugar levels, a result of disruption in the mechanism that allows the body's cells to convert blood sugar (glucose) into usable energy. Under normal conditions the pancreas regulates blood sugar; its beta cells secrete a hormone called insulin, which regulates sugar metabolism. People with Type One or juvenile-onset diabetes, the kind that usually begins in childhood, do not produce insulin at all. People with Type Two or adult-onset diabetes, the most common form (9 out of 10 cases), usually found in people over 40, can produce the hormone but have a resistance to insulin or poor utilization of it.

Most cases of diabetes are thought to be the result of a genetic disorder. Type One diabetes is usually sudden in onset with severe symptoms. Type Two tends to be variable in onset (slow or sudden) and symptoms can vary in their intensity.

In either case, the symptoms may include increased urination and thirst, tiredness, blurred vision, weight loss, infection, and numbness and burning in the hands and feet. In severe cases symptoms such as nausea, vomiting, stomach cramps, deep and rapid breathing, a fruity breath odor, and ultimately coma and death may occur.

Diabetes has no cure, but treatment is well known and generally effective. Type One cases require insulin injections. Type Two cases may be treated with oral hypoglycemic agents and sometimes require insulin injections.

Advances in medical technology have made diabetes a manageable illness. Yet even with the availability of insulin therapy, diabetics still can exert a significant impact on their health through the food choices they make. Doctors usually offer some guidelines, but diabetics can also benefit from more comprehensive sources of information about ways to make eating a satisfying as well as a health-promoting experience. The following book is one such source.

THE UCSD HEALTHY DIET FOR DIABETES: A COMPREHENSIVE NUTRITIONAL GUIDE AND COOKBOOK

by Susan Algert, M.S., R.D.,
Barbara Grasse, R.D., C.D.E. and
Annie Durning, M.S., R.D.
Houghton Mifflin Company
Boston: 1990

ABOUT THE AUTHORS Susan Algert holds a master's degree in nutrition and has been a research dietitian at the General Clinical Research Center, University of California at San Diego (UCSD) Medical Center, for seven years. Prior to this she held the same position at the Oregon Health Sciences University.

Barbara Grasse has worked for 10 years as a research dietitian at UCSD and is currently the senior research dietitian there. She holds a Certified Diabetes Educator degree and a master's in nutrition.

Annie Durning has worked for six years as a research dietitian for UCSD and holds a master's degree in nutrition.

OVERVIEW Based upon the nutritional/medical research into diabetes conducted at the UCSD General Clinical Research Center, this book aims to give the diabetic specific dietary guidelines as well as a large number of choices within those guidelines. The book contains 225 recipes, including ethnic cuisines such as Chinese, Mexican, French, German, Italian, Indian, Middle Eastern, Far Eastern, and South American, as well as vegetarian dishes, all modified to meet the nutritional needs of diabetics. The dietary focus in all recipes is on complex carbohydrates, such as rice, beans, and pasta, avoiding refined sugars, and using meat as a condiment rather than main ingredient.

The book follows the nutritional guidelines of the American Diabetic Association, which include maintaining appropriate levels of glucose and fat in the bloodstream; eating consistently (approximately the same time and amount each day); managing weight; limiting salt, sugar, fat, and alcohol, while increasing consumption of complex carbohydrates within specified goals; consuming adequate amounts of fiber; and reducing saturated fat and cholesterol while increasing polyunsaturated and monounsaturated fats.

The authors give advice on identifying and avoiding hidden sugars and salt and replacing them with healthful substitutes. They set reasonable limits on refined sugars, sodium, and alcohol, backing up these restrictions with sobering scientific data—something physicians don't always have time to do.

The UCSD Healthy Diet also discusses the nutritional insurance of vitamin and mineral supplements and the pros and cons of artificial and other sweeteners. Fructose, for example, is a healthful sweetener that will not elevate blood sugar any more than complex carbohydrates do—yet high-fructose corn syrup contains glucose and *will* raise blood sugar.

Another important topic the authors cover is weight control. In addition to being a primary cause of Type Two diabetes, obesity also greatly increases the risks associated with diabetes. They point out that weight loss and maintenance are crucial and that even a 10 percent weight reduction can make a considerable difference. The authors also make important distinctions about the nature of excess weight. Upper-body obesity, for example, is most often associated with diabetes.

The authors recommend the use of a food diary along with behavioral modification, exercise, and a social support group. They give specific advice about all of these components. Tips for dining out and special occasions encompass ethnic as well as continental eateries and fast food; they include restaurant selection, ways to reduce fat in restaurant meals, and advice about making necessary adjustments to other meals during the day in order to compensate for special-occasion meals.

Throughout the book the authors emphasize the theme of give-and-take. They recommend calorie counting but permit food exchanges that allow flexibility within safe guidelines.

They also provide extensive instructions for self-monitoring of blood-sugar levels as part of a comprehensive approach to working with your physician to control diabetes. Advice includes what to do when you get sick, since having the flu or a serious cold can be especially hard on diabetics.

NUTRITIONAL EVALUATION An analysis of one day's sample menus found the calories about 300 below the book's own recommendation, but still within a safe and healthful range. These calories break down as follows:

Carbohydrates 53%
Protein 20%
Fat 27%
Sodium .... 2,307 milligrams
Fiber .... 24 grams
Cholesterol .... 155 milligrams

The major nutrient breakdown is within a few percentage points of the authors' recommendations (complex carbohydrates 55 percent, protein 20 percent, fat 25 percent), but not entirely in line with current health goals (complex carbohydrates 55 percent, protein 15 percent, fat 30 percent or less). Protein is a little on the high side, but with carbohydrates comprising over 50 percent and fat below 30 percent, I feel that the protein level is reasonable. Cholesterol and sodium are within recommended maximums and fiber is well above the recommended minimum.

All essential vitamins and minerals meet 100 percent of the RDA except for thiamine and niacin, which exceed the acceptable two-thirds of the recommendations. An increase in whole grains and vegetables should increase those two nutrients as well as favorably adjust the carbohydrate/protein/fat ratio.

PRACTICALITY Many of the recipes are quick to make; about a third are microwaveable and can be prepared in under half an hour. All of the menus come with nutritional breakdowns to assist in the otherwise arduous task of record keeping. Adherence to this diet also requires some degree of calculation and may be difficult at first, but keeping track of sugar and food intake is essential in coping with diabetes. After a while most diabetics should be able to master the food exchange system and make short work of it.

Although the diet is flexible and accommodates eating out, it does require a good deal of planning and adjusting of other snacks and meals during that day. This, again, is a reality of diabetes. For special occasions, the recipes include dishes that the diabetic can eat along with everyone else.

Although refined sugars are not recommended for diabetics, this diet does allow limited quantities and also gives advice about wine selection for those special occasions.

ANALYSIS OF 1-DAY MENU FOR MALE, AGE 35

The UCSD Healthy Diet for Diabetes

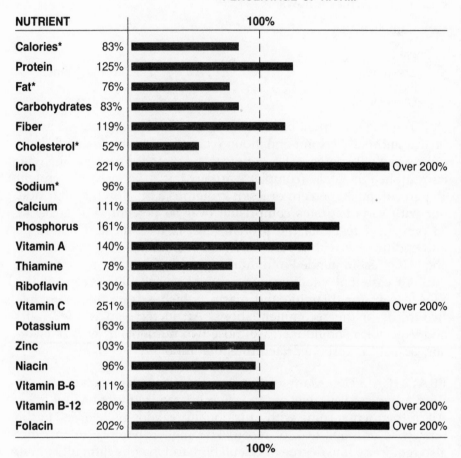

NUTRIENT		PERCENTAGE OF RA/RM 100%
Calories*	83%	
Protein	125%	
Fat*	76%	
Carbohydrates	83%	
Fiber	119%	
Cholesterol*	52%	
Iron	221%	Over 200%
Sodium*	96%	
Calcium	111%	
Phosphorus	161%	
Vitamin A	140%	
Thiamine	78%	
Riboflavin	130%	
Vitamin C	251%	Over 200%
Potassium	163%	
Zinc	103%	
Niacin	96%	
Vitamin B-6	111%	
Vitamin B-12	280%	Over 200%
Folacin	202%	Over 200%

100%

*Recommended maximum allowance. Nutrient should not exceed 100%.

An important aspect of this diet is that it can accommodate diabetic children who must monitor sugar intake but still need enough calories to ensure normal growth.

LIFESTYLE AND EXERCISE The entire book is really a course in behavior modification for the diabetic. The book teaches ways to change your lifestyle in order to accommodate the limitations set by this disease.

The book recommends a physician's approval before beginning a program of aerobic exercise, the intensity level to be geared toward the individual, whether sedentary or fairly active. Special consideration is given to insulin-dependent diabetics, whose exercise duration must be coordinated with insulin dosages. Overall, the authors warn against excessive exercise for any diabetic. Otherwise, the authors strongly advocate exercise for several reasons. Exercise can help control diabetes, especially Type Two, since it encourages weight control and increases the sensitivity of body cells to insulin so that they can better utilize it. Exercise also improves cardiovascular fitness and self-image.

WHY IT WORKS   This book gives the diabetic some tools to implement healthy living principles and is an excellent resource and workbook. The recipes dispel the myth equating diabetic diets with culinary blandness, boredom, and deprivation. In particular, the use of herbs and spices provides low-sodium, low-refined-sugar foods that really taste good. This nutritional guide and cookbook contains many usable charts and tables and a lot of valuable advice that can have a meaningful impact on the quality of life for the diabetic.

Perhaps most important, the authors address diabetes not as an isolated health problem with isolated solutions, but place it in the context of overall good health—no sense managing one illness at the expense of bringing on another. Their message is that you can be diabetic and still live a full and enjoyable life while keeping your blood sugar under control.

POTENTIAL DRAWBACKS   The only criticism I have of this book concerns a few relatively minor factual errors. The authors describe "8 essential amino acids out of a total of 22" (there are actually 9 essentials out of 23). They erroneously lump all shellfish together as having higher cholesterol than fish. While this is accurate for lobster, crab, and shrimp, it is not so for surf clams or sea scallops.

SECOND OPINIONS   ". . . offers sensible, authoritative, and practical information for diabetics, and can be used as guide to healthy living by nondiabetics as well."

—Library Journal

"As the authors—dieticians at the University of California at San Diego Medical Center—show, diabetic meals do not have to be dreary. . . . They set nutritional goals for diabetics and dispense essential advice in a friendly tone."

—Publishers Weekly

MEDICAL/HEALTH/SPECIALTY DIETS

FOOD ALLERGIES

ABOUT 35 MILLION AMERICANS—17 percent of the population—are estimated to have some kind of allergy. Many of them suffer from food-related allergies, although the precise number is not known.

While the Asthma and Allergy Foundation of America sets the figure at about one million people, physicians who specialize in allergies explain that it is difficult to determine the number because food-allergy tests are not as reliable as other allergy tests, nor are patients themselves an accurate guide. For example, many who claim to be food-allergic do not understand that lactose intolerance and wheat intolerance are not allergies (see those sections for further information). On the other hand, many people who suffer food-allergy symptoms never seek medical treatment. Of course, what matters most is whether *you* have a food allergy, diagnosed or undiagnosed.

When you consume a food that you are allergic to, your immune system identifies the unfriendly invader and dispenses antibodies to destroy or neutralize it. These antibodies are produced by special cells called plasma cells or B cells located in bone marrow, lymph nodes, and in the mucosal lining of the respiratory, gastrointestinal, and genital tracts.

The body stores many of these antibodies in much the same way armies stockpile weapons, in anticipation of the next invasion. The body can normally deal with small doses of invaders—in fact, it does so daily—but the continued consumption of an allergenic substance can overstimulate the antibodies, instigating adverse symptoms. These symptoms can include headaches, a stuffy nose, sinus problems, canker sores, sore throat, swollen glands, a persistent cough, asthma, heart palpitations, episodes of alternating tension and fatigue, muscular chest pains, heartburn, acid indigestion, stomach pain, cramps, bloating, diarrhea, constipation, urinary frequency, urinary burning and hesitancy, vaginal irritation, rectal itching, arthritis, joint stiffness and swelling, psoriasis, hives, itching, and welts.

The foods most commonly associated with allergenic reactions include citrus fruits, corn, chicken, oats, eggs, soy, vinegar and other fermented products (such as wine, beer, and yeast), coffee, tea, cane sugar, chocolate, tomatoes, peas, peanuts, and onions and chives. There are numerous other possible culprits.

Food allergies are, for the most part, incurable. They are, however, manageable—but only if you identify which food(s) you are allergic to. The following book offers a method for doing so.

The Allergy Discovery Diet: A Rotation Diet for Discovering Your Allergies to Food

by John E. Postley, M.D.
Recipes by Janet M. Barton
Doubleday
New York: 1990

ABOUT THE AUTHOR Dr. John Postley is a New York City allergist specializing in the treatment of adult asthma. He is an assistant clinical professor of medicine at Columbia University. Janet Barton has a master's degree in special education from American University.

OVERVIEW The book's purpose is to help people with undiagnosed symptoms determine if those symptoms are due to food allergies and, if so, what food or foods are responsible. According to the author, food allergies are impossible to predict. There are no equations such as "allergy to corn = asthma." Any food allergy can cause any symptoms. There are no medical tests to accurately identify food allergies, claims Dr. Postley. He discovered this firsthand when his wife experienced severe symptoms that puzzled her doctor. Postley took it upon himself to determine whether she was suffering a food allergy, and out of his research and experimentation he not only solved the mystery of her symptoms—the problems turned out to be an intolerance to dairy products and an allergy to chocolate—but also designed a program for others to use.

The two-phase, three-week diet is a personalized and scientifically organized program of over 400 recipes using common foods. *Phase I: Elimination* is designed to enable you to purge your body of the suspected allergenic food and to confirm that your symptoms are, in fact, the result of a food allergy. During this phase you eat only hypoallergenic foods—those foods that, based upon documented medical research, are considered least likely to cause allergic reactions. These include tapioca, beef, lamb, veal, rice, lentils, pears, squash, olive oil, cucumbers, potatoes, and bananas.

In addition to avoiding hyperallergenic foods (those *most* likely to cause allergic reactions), you are instructed to cease medications (with your physician's prior approval) and vitamin and mineral supplements. Fresh fruits and vegetables are emphasized to ensure an adequate supply of natural nutrients in their place. This phase can last up to 15 days.

Phase II: Reintroduction is designed to pinpoint the food culprit by isolating it. This is done by reexposing yourself to small amounts of various foods, rotating them, and monitoring yourself for the recurrence of symptoms. During this phase, which lasts about two weeks, you eat only unprocessed, single-ingredient foods, not repeating any food within any three-day period. Each day of the diet is presented as a self-contained unit with lists of permissible foods, menus, and accompanying recipes.

Postley provides tips on how to maintain a detailed food diary in order to match symptoms with hyperallegenic foods. He furnishes comprehensive lists and descriptions of the most common hyperallergenic foods along with a discussion of hidden sources of them in processed foods.

If symptoms persist after you have carefully followed Phase II for two weeks, you can rule out a food allergy as the culprit, according to Postley.

NUTRITIONAL EVALUATION   Analysis was done of a two-day average of the Elimination Phase, which can last up to 15 days and is thus the part of the diet you will spend the majority of your time on. (Phase II varies from day to day and from individual to individual and would thus be impossible to analyze in this manner).

For some people, the calories are a little low for a diet not intended for weight loss, but an extra serving from the recommended food list each day could remedy that. Calories break down as follows:

```
Carbohydrates ........................... 47%
Protein .................................. 14%
Fat ...................................... 39%
Sodium ................................... 1,304 milligrams
Fiber .................................... 25 grams
Cholesterol .............................. 116 milligrams
```

ANALYSIS OF 2-DAY MENU FOR FEMALE, AGE 35

The Allergy Discovery Diet

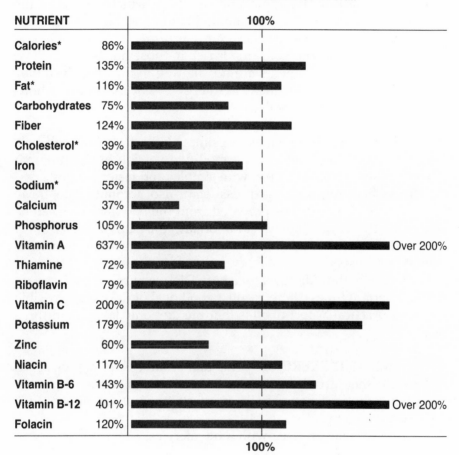

PERCENTAGE OF RA/RM

NUTRIENT		100%
Calories*	86%	
Protein	135%	
Fat*	116%	
Carbohydrates	75%	
Fiber	124%	
Cholesterol*	39%	
Iron	86%	
Sodium*	55%	
Calcium	37%	
Phosphorus	105%	
Vitamin A	637%	Over 200%
Thiamine	72%	
Riboflavin	79%	
Vitamin C	200%	
Potassium	179%	
Zinc	60%	
Niacin	117%	
Vitamin B-6	143%	
Vitamin B-12	401%	Over 200%
Folacin	120%	

100%

*Recommended maximum allowance. Nutrient should not exceed 100%.

Protein is within established health goals. Carbohydrates, however, are low, and fat is significantly higher than recommended maximums. Even if it is not intended to promote weight loss, any diet concerned with good health should closely conform to established goals. Increasing complex carbohydrates and decreasing fat consumption should enable you to make necessary adjustments without deviating significantly from the prescribed eating plan.

Fiber is a healthful 25 milligrams, and sodium and cholesterol are both below recommended maximums.

All essential vitamins and minerals meet 100 percent of the RDA except for iron, thiamine, and riboflavin which do exceed the acceptable two-thirds of the recommendation and calcium and zinc which do not. These deficiencies are due primarily to the elimination of certain hyperallergenic foods rich in those nutrients.

Nutritional supplements are not allowed in this diet since they too can be allergenic, but since the Allergy Discovery Diet is a short-term plan, this is not likely to present any serious concern.

PRACTICALITY   The recipes are simple, easy to follow, and provide variety. Postley also offers a modified version of the program (Diet Express) for busy people, with simpler and faster recipes.

This diet—regular or express—can also accommodate travel and dining out. The dishes prepared from the book's recipes can be served to the entire family. Additionally, the author spells out a modified version of this diet for parents to administer to their children if they suspect a food allergy.

Although the Allergy Discovery Diet requires eating certain foods at certain times, there is still a good deal of flexibility. Possibly the most practical aspect of all is that the diet only lasts about three weeks.

LIFESTYLE AND EXERCISE   This diet assumes a strong desire to isolate and then avoid the allergenic substance(s). Considering the potential symptoms of food allergy reactions, motivation shouldn't be hard to come by.

Exercise is not an issue with food allergies.

WHY IT WORKS   Though not a new idea, this elimination diet is comprehensive and easy to follow. Diagnosing an allergy is like detective work, and this diet gives a framework for conducting an investigation. Of course, not everyone who thinks he or she has a food allergy actually has one. But even if the diet only serves to rule out such allergies, the experience can prove to be a positive one. Learning your responses to various foods and becoming an expert in label reading can help in achieving and maintaining overall health in the long run.

The food plans allow three meals plus snacks and desserts to ensure satisfaction. The book is easy to read; it is filled with interesting case histories of people with a wide variety of food allergies.

POTENTIAL DRAWBACKS   Postley does not provide specific portion size recommendations because this is not a weight loss diet. But many people, overweight or not, need some boundaries as to portion size, and so it might have been better to give optional guidelines.

SECOND OPINION   "For the most part, the authors argue the case convincingly [that food sensitivities are responsible for many chronic conditions with no other apparent medical causes]. Yet they do not consider the problem of people suffering from chronic conditions not helped by the exclusion of such foods."

—Publishers Weekly

MEDICAL/HEALTH/SPECIALTY DIETS

HYPERTENSION

THIS IS THE MEDICAL TERM for high blood pressure, a condition in which the heart has to pump harder than normal because of an excess of fluid in the bloodstream combined with narrowed or constricted arteries. It is called the silent killer because it may be asymptomatic for many years but can eventually cause heart failure, kidney disease, stroke, and blindness—so if you've been diagnosed as hypertensive, consider yourself fortunate to know that you can do something about the condition. Dietary considerations along with physical activity can play a significant part. The following book offers help.

RECIPES FOR THE HEART: A NUTRITIONAL GUIDE FOR PEOPLE WITH HIGH BLOOD PRESSURE

by Lucy M. Williams, M.S., M.Ed., R.D.
Sandridge Publishing
Bowling Green, Ohio: 1990

ABOUT THE AUTHOR Williams received her M.S. from Indiana University and her M.Ed. from Bowling Green University. She is a licensed dietitian, a member of the American Dietetic Association, and a nutritional consultant and teacher in Bowling Green, Ohio.

OVERVIEW The goal of this book is to help the reader understand high blood pressure and the dietary changes required to control it. Williams describes the cause and treatment of hypertension and enumerates the role of nutrition in that treatment. She describes the nutrients vital to controlling blood pressure and suggests the best ways to get them—complete with food source lists, food content lists, and recipes high in those needed nutrients.

Since coping with hypertension is as much about what *not* to eat as about what *to* eat, the author also discusses the problems with sodium and fat and limits them in her food selection and recipe suggestions. The discussion of sodium is particularly in-depth and deals not only with its biochemistry, but also with the behavioral aspects of dietary modification. Williams advises, for example, to taste food before salting. She discusses ways to make food choices low in fat and to turn bad eating habits into good ones.

This is primarily a recipe book, and its focus is on cooking methods that will promote blood pressure control. The recipes, thus, are high in potassium, calcium, and carbohydrates and low in fat and sodium. The 83 recipes include beverages, breads, desserts, fruit dishes, meats and other main dishes, sauces and dressings, soups, and vegetable dishes. Microwaveable recipes are provided to replace prepackaged microwaveable foods, many of which are deleterious to anyone with high blood pressure.

Though not a weight loss book, *Recipes for the Heart* does conform to national guidelines for weight loss—and for good reason: obesity is a major cause and complicating factor in hypertension.

NUTRITIONAL EVALUATION   This is primarily a recipe book with no formal menus. Thus, I selected a typical day's eating plan from among the recipes, using standard serving sizes. Analysis found calories within an acceptable range, but remember that this assumes moderate portion size.

Carbohydrates 55%
Protein 12%
Fat 33%
Sodium . . . . 1,867 milligrams
Fiber . . . . 12 grams
Cholesterol . . . . 107 milligrams

Protein, carbohydrates, cholesterol, and sodium are all within recommended goals. Fat is high, but it should be noted that the author does provide low-fat substitutions for high-fat food choices. Fiber is low, but the author does stress the use of fresh fruits and vegetables.

Essential micronutrients meet or exceed 100 percent of the RDA except for vitamin C, folacin, and thiamine, which exceed two-thirds of the RDA, and niacin, iron, and zinc, which do not.

PRACTICALITY   Home cooking can be somewhat time consuming, but this book addresses that concern with a number of fast and simple recipes. The book is easy to read, with helpful charts and lists and a comprehensive recipe index for quick and easy access.

LIFESTYLE AND EXERCISE   Although this is a cookbook, it does address what I consider to be an important behavioral aspect: the act of cooking, making *preparation* as much a part of eating as the actual consumption of food. This can do wonders toward altering your eating habits. Additionally, the author suggests keeping a food diary, but only for the first two or three days to get on the right track.

The book encourages walking and other activity but does not give any specific exercise advice.

WHY IT WORKS   The book stresses an individualized approach to hypertension management—finding your own way within the broad guidelines and suggestions. These suggestions are comprehensive and include many things that hypertensive patients are not always aware of—for example, that sodium substitutes may not be a healthful alternative for everyone (some of them contain aluminum

ANALYSIS OF 1-DAY MENU FOR FEMALE, AGE 35

Recipes for the Heart

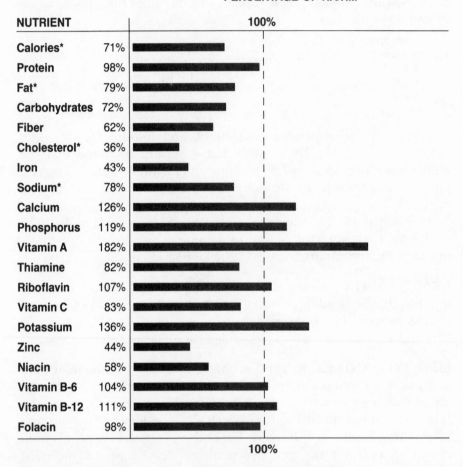

NUTRIENT		PERCENTAGE OF RA/RM
Calories*	71%	
Protein	98%	
Fat*	79%	
Carbohydrates	72%	
Fiber	62%	
Cholesterol*	36%	
Iron	43%	
Sodium*	78%	
Calcium	126%	
Phosphorus	119%	
Vitamin A	182%	
Thiamine	82%	
Riboflavin	107%	
Vitamin C	83%	
Potassium	136%	
Zinc	44%	
Niacin	58%	
Vitamin B-6	104%	
Vitamin B-12	111%	
Folacin	98%	

100%

*Recommended maximum allowance. Nutrient should not exceed 100%.

or potassium, either of which can cause health problems if used in excess).

With the sometimes deceptive packaging practices of some food manufacturers, hypertensives need to know not only how to cut down on salt but also how to avoid hidden sources of sodium through overall awareness and a trained eye at label reading. The words "low sodium" on a packaged food do not necessarily mean that the sodium content conforms to health goals. To take the awareness model one step further, the recipes within the book give clear nutritional information.

This author simplifies a good deal of somewhat complex medical information and makes it accessible with clear illustrative tables and charts. She also admits the limitations of this—or, for that matter, *any*—book by recommending not only the supervision of a physician but also the advice of a registered dietitian to ensure a well-balanced diet program. She provides a useful list of additional literature on hypertension.

POTENTIAL DRAWBACKS As I have discovered with many books, this one fails to distinguish adequately between polyunsaturated and monounsaturated oils, potentially leaving readers believing they are healthily equivalent when they are not.

By its own admission, this book may not, by itself, be enough to inspire the lifestyle changes necessary to manage hypertension. For many people, however, it can be a valuable tool to be used along with medical supervision, a support group, an exercise program, and an R.D.

SECOND OPINION "If hypertension is a particular concern of yours, you'll want this new book. . . . In addition to recipes, it discusses cause and control of hypertension, and includes fast food facts, weight control tips and charts of common food sources of sodium, potassium, and calcium."

—*Lowfat Lifeline Newsletter*

MEDICAL/HEALTH/SPECIALTY DIETS

HYPOGLYCEMIA

HYPOGLYCEMIA IS THE FLIP side of diabetes: a condition of low blood sugar resulting from an overproduction—rather than underproduction—of insulin by the pancreas. When a person with hypoglycemia eats sugar, the pancreas overreacts, releasing so much insulin that it lowers blood sugar to a point considerably below normal. This in turn can trigger a hunger sensation and the desire for a fast glucose (sugar) fix, such as a candy bar, soda, or other food high in sugar. This, in turn, will cause the pancreas to release even more insulin, producing an ongoing blood sugar roller coaster.

Symptoms include weakness, fatigue, malaise, restlessness, irritability, profuse sweating, dizziness, trembling, blurred vision, slurred speech, tingling in the lips or hands, and headaches. In severe cases, hypoglycemics can suffer mental disturbances, delirium, coma, and even death.

In many cases, hypoglycemia can be treated through hormone therapy and/or careful dietary practices and monitoring. Obviously, medical supervision is needed in dealing with such a serious illness, but greater understanding can enable the patient to fully participate in his or her own treatment. The following book can provide that understanding.

THE DO'S AND DON'TS OF LOW BLOOD SUGAR

by Roberta Ruggiero
Frederick Fell Publishers, Inc.
Hollywood, Florida: 1988

ABOUT THE AUTHOR   Ruggiero is founder and president of the Hypoglycemic Research Foundation, Inc., a support group that holds monthly meetings featuring educational talks from health professionals. A hypoglycemic herself, Ruggiero has utilized her experiences along with 10 years of research and involvement with experts in the field in writing this book to help others avoid her own unpleasant experiences and to give support, encouragement, and easy-to-follow guidelines for coping with hypoglycemia.

OVERVIEW   Ruggiero begins by setting hypoglycemia within a historical framework, opening with the medical community's recognition of hypoglycemia as a disease in 1949, and continuing through the 1970s, when it became a "trendy" disease (at the same time as the AMA inexplicably labeled hypoglycemia a nondisease), right up to the present in which conflict and confusion about hypoglycemia persist.

Given this climate of relative chaos, the author presents some helpful do's and don'ts for selecting the best doctor and for getting the most out of that physician. She reminds the reader that even a very good physician is only as good as the cooperation and participation from the patient. She cites the current morass of contradictions in the medical community over the proper diet for hypoglycemics. Some say high protein, others say high complex carbohydrates. Who is right? According to Ruggiero, no one and everyone. As a hypoglycemic, she contends, you must find your own individualized diet to meet the unique needs of your body.

The author recommends trial and error as the means to achieving a customized hypoglycemic diet. She suggests one to ten days of keeping a diary of food eaten and medications taken. When symptoms occur, you identify what food you most recently ate and eliminate it from your diet. If you believe that medicines are responsible for your symptoms, Ruggiero suggests contacting the prescribing physician.

The book lists the most likely culprits in the cause and symptoms of hypoglycemia: refined sugars, white flour, alcohol, caffeine, and tobacco. She does not, however, recommend immediately withdrawing any of them. Rather, she advises a strategy of gradual reduction and eventual elimination.

The *Do's and Don'ts of Low Blood Sugar* provides reasonable and healthful alternatives to a number of potentially offending foods, along with advice on identifying and avoiding hidden sugars in processed and other foods. This program has the potential of leading the hypoglycemic to a wholesome way of eating that will not only decrease the risk of hypoglycemic symptoms but improve overall health and well-being. Ruggiero recommends vitamin and mineral supplementation to ensure adequate nutrition.

Hypoglycemia is more than a disease of food selection; its treatment requires dietary modifications in a variety of ways. *The Do's and Dont's* includes advice about when to eat, how often to eat, how much water to drink (hypoglycemics need adequate fluid even more urgently than do others), how to rotate foods to avoid food sensitivity, how to prepare foods, and even when to seek psychotherapy as a part of treatment.

According to its author, this book is only the beginning. She provides a reading list and urges readers to pursue a fuller awareness of their illness in order to minimize its effects.

NUTRITIONAL EVALUATION   I prepared a daily menu from the suggested breakfasts, lunches, dinners, and snacks provided in the book. I used standard serving sizes where none were specified by the author, which may account for why the calories came in a little on the low side. Those calories average out to this approximate breakdown:

Carbohydrates	52%
Protein	34%
Fat	14%
Sodium	1,983 milligrams
Fiber	24 grams
Cholesterol	408 milligrams

Protein and cholesterol are both too high—in part because I selected a recommended breakfast that included an egg. Assuming

ANALYSIS OF 1-DAY MENU FOR FEMALE, AGE 35

The Do's and Don'ts of Low Blood Sugar

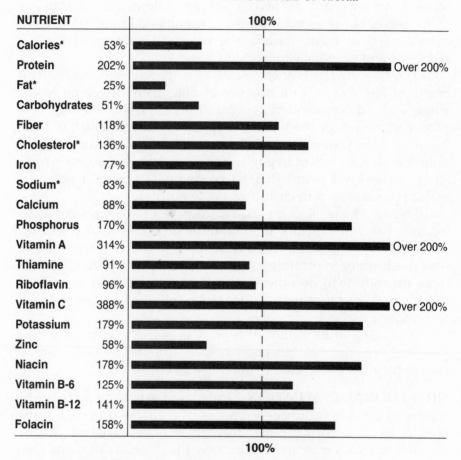

PERCENTAGE OF RA/RM

NUTRIENT		100%
Calories*	53%	
Protein	202%	Over 200%
Fat*	25%	
Carbohydrates	51%	
Fiber	118%	
Cholesterol*	136%	
Iron	77%	
Sodium*	83%	
Calcium	88%	
Phosphorus	170%	
Vitamin A	314%	Over 200%
Thiamine	91%	
Riboflavin	96%	
Vitamin C	388%	Over 200%
Potassium	179%	
Zinc	58%	
Niacin	178%	
Vitamin B-6	125%	
Vitamin B-12	141%	
Folacin	158%	

100%

*Recommended maximum allowance. Nutrient should not exceed 100%.

you do not repeat the same breakfast every day and in general use the suggested meal plans to eat a variety of foods, the protein and cholesterol levels should decrease over the course of a week. Carbohydrates are a little low, but do meet the pre-1989 RDA goals that were current when this book was written. Fiber and sodium both fall within recommended ranges.

Essential micronutrients meet or exceed 100 percent of the RDA, except for iron, calcium, thiamine, and riboflavin, all of which are above two-thirds of the RDA, and zinc, which is not. An increase in whole-grain products and the inclusion of seafood will increase zinc intake.

PRACTICALITY   By nature, hypoglycemia is an illness of *im*practicality. Having to eat six small meals per day and always carry emergency food around are among its potential inconveniences. Ruggiero's advice is an attempt to reduce those inconveniences and help readers accept them.

LIFESTYLE AND EXERCISE   While neither a psychiatric nor behavioral specialist, the author nevertheless makes clear the acute importance of lifestyle modification in blood-sugar management. Her suggestions include membership in Overeaters Anonymous— or even in Alcoholics Anonymous—for those who feel they are addicted to refined sugars and starches and need group support. In general, she promotes an ever-expanding knowledge of hypoglycemia and its treatments.

The author also recommends positive-thinking self-help books as part of the behavioral approach, along with her own behavioral tips, to help hypoglycemics change their concept not only of meals and snacks but, more important, to change their concept of *self*. "Don't compare your results to those of others," she implores. Everyone's metabolism is different.

The program stresses the importance of daily exercise, suggesting a walking program with some do's and don'ts for hypoglycemics:

• Do get medical approval.

• Do eat one hour before exercising to avoid a drop in blood sugar and dizziness.

• Do stretch correctly before exercising, and cool down afterwards.

• Don't set high expectations.

• Don't think you can lose weight quickly by pushing yourself to exercise too frequently.

• Don't exercise on a full stomach.

- Don't push yourself to exercise if you are too fatigued or experiencing symptoms.

- Don't compare your progress with someone else's.

- Don't give up too quickly on any program because you don't see results.

WHY IT WORKS   The author underscores the importance of self-education about hypoglycemia as the cornerstone of controlling the symptoms and managing the illness. Blood-sugar illnesses are, by and large, manageable but delicate, and awareness is a key to health and well-being.

Ruggiero does not pretend that this book or any other book could be a panacea for the hypoglycemic. She advises the hypoglycemic to seek the advice of an M.D. well-versed in nutrition or the advice of an R.D. in concert with a physician. The suggestions and information in this book can help hypoglycemics get the most benefit from consulting those health professionals.

The narrative is fast, easy reading with a positive and reassuring tone. Perhaps the most valuable element of this book is the personal experience and firsthand knowledge conveyed by the author.

POTENTIAL DRAWBACKS   Advising hypoglycemics addicted to sugar to seek help at OA or AA may not be suitable for some, particularly those addictive personalities who need professional therapy. Ruggiero does not make this distinction.

While the author's overall emphasis on knowledge and self-awareness is sensible, the suggestion to weigh yourself daily as a part of that awareness may be excessive. Daily weight fluctuations may be more deceptive than enlightening and can create anxiety and/or frustration. Weighing-in once or twice a week should be sufficient.

Finally, the exercise advice is a bit sketchy. Although the author stresses its importance, she does not devote an appropriate amount of attention to it.

SECOND OPINION   "This is a very reasonable, well-researched presentation of a topic which has often been treated faddishly in other publications."

—Library Journal

MEDICAL/HEALTH/SPECIALTY DIETS

INFLAMMATORY BOWEL DISEASE (I.B.D.)

THIS ILLNESS, WHICH CURRENTLY affects between 500,000 and 800,000 adults and children in the United States alone, is a chronic inflammatory disease of the intestinal tract (the bowel wall), sometimes involving lesions. It can vary in intensity and in location. When it strikes the ileim (the last portion of the small intestine), it is known as ileitis; when it strikes the large intestine (colon) it is known as ulcerative colitis. Crohn's disease, or regional ileitis, can strike anywhere along the digestive tract from the esophagus to the colon. Inflammatory bowel disease is the category under which all of these conditions fall.

Common symptoms include diarrhea, abdominal pain, weight loss, growth failure in children, rectal bleeding (which can lead to anemia), and poor food absorption (which can lead to malnutrition). Severe flare-ups of I.B.D. can require hospitalization. Not all symptoms occur in the intestinal tract. Mouth ulcers, joint inflammation, and the appearance of red nodules on the skin can also result from I.B.D. flare-ups.

The causes of this illness are unknown. Men and women seem equally vulnerable, but I.B.D. does run in families. We do not know if that is because of heredity or shared environmental factors. Most I.B.D. sufferers are between the ages of 12 and 40, and most of them experience their first symptoms before age 15. A great number describe themselves as being unable to deal well with stress, but researchers do not believe that I.B.D. is the result of emotional stress. Rather, they believe that stress aggravates the disease.

There is no known cure. Medical intervention is meant to reduce the symptoms only. Sometimes surgery is prescribed, but such measures do not ensure the end of suffering. The best therapy for this disease is a prudent and balanced diet avoiding known troublesome foods, along with stress management and an appropriate exercise program. The following book makes such recommendations.

Eating Right for a Bad Gut (The Complete Nutritional Guide to Ileitus, Colitis, Crohn's Disease, and Inflammatory Bowel Disease)

by James Scala, Ph.D.
Penguin Books
New York: 1990

ABOUT THE AUTHOR   Dr. Scala has been involved in nutrition and health research for more than 20 years. A graduate of Cornell University with a doctoral degree in biochemistry, he has taught nutrition/biochemistry at Georgetown Medical School, the University of Oklahoma Medical School, Ohio College of Medicine, and the University of California at Berkeley. He is an elected member of the American Dietetic Association, the American Institute of Nutrition, the American College of Nutrition, and the British Nutrition Society. His previous books include *The Arthritis Relief Diet* (see earlier section in this book) and *The High Blood Pressure Relief Diet*.

OVERVIEW   Scala's stated goals in this book are to "help sufferers [of I.B.D.] learn how to identify foods and other things that cause flare-ups" and "to help keep foods that cause flare-ups to a minimum." Scala cites scientific evidence to support his belief that dietary modifications can greatly reduce and control the symptoms of I.B.D.

After providing an overview of the workings of the digestive tract and the nature of this disease, he gives some general eating guidelines for people with I.B.D. with two important objectives in mind: (1) avoid flare-ups, and (2) ensure adequate nutrition in the face of potential malabsorption problems.

These goals are based upon a nutrient breakdown of 50–60 percent complex carbohydrates, 10–15 percent protein, and less than 30 percent fat. [*Editor's Note: these are slightly different from the goals used throughout this book.*] Scala gives a thorough review of the nutritional aspects of I.B.D. in relation to these macronutrients— incomplete versus complete proteins, good versus bad fats, complex versus simple carbohydrates, and hard versus soft water. He advises the avoidance of empty-calorie foods in particular and processed foods in general, in favor of natural sources of nutrition, and he provides an in-depth discussion of the importance of dietary fiber to I.B.D. sufferers.

Since dietary fiber can be as much a problem to people with I.B.D. as a help, Scala gives specific advice about how to ensure that fiber can be easily digested to enhance intestinal health. He recommends 30 grams of fiber per day and describes what he calls the "fiber matrix," his rules about fiber. For example, the peels of many fruits and vegetables need to be removed and insoluble fiber sources must be cooked until tender. Scala also discusses diverticulosis, an illness of the large intestine, and its relationship to fiber. He recommends fiber supplements and suggests ways to minimize their potential side effects.

Addressing specific measures for preventing I.B.D. flare-ups, Scala lists foods to avoid (such as alcohol, chocolate, and refined sugars) along with label-reading advice to identify hidden sources of them. He recommends keeping a food diary, eating frequent small meals, and chewing thoroughly. Scala offers advice for preventing specific kinds of flare-ups, such as diarrhea. He lists foods to stay away from as well as foods to emphasize, and discusses some interesting folk remedies for certain symptoms.

Since, according to Scala, I.B.D. is often associated with lactose intolerance and other food intolerances and allergies, he offers advice about how to conduct an elimination diet under the guidance of your physician.

Painful flare-ups are not the only serious problems I.B.D. sufferers must cope with: the disease can cause the malabsorption of important nutrients. Scala discusses this problem and offers advice about nutritional supplementation. He recommends a multiple vitamin and mineral supplement along with extra calcium, iron, and zinc to compensate for the increased energy needs and elevated metabolism associated with the diseased state. The author details the important vitamins and minerals and their roles in relation to overall body functioning and I.B.D. (for example, potassium can be depleted by diarrhea). He also advises a balanced predigested food supplement such as Criticare (Bristol-Meyers) or Vital (Ross Labs) to help rest the bowels during flare-ups.

Scala addresses being underweight, a problem many I.B.D. patients face. He explains the most common reasons: malabsorption due to inflammation, nutrient loss due to diarrhea, and loss of appetite due to discomfort. He suggests supplementary foods that counteract these problems without putting demands on the intestines—foods such as shakes, prepared drinks, and puddings, which deliver calories, protein, vitamins and minerals, and a balance of sodium and potassium. He suggests overall guidelines for gaining weight through increased lean body mass rather than fat, but cautions against doing so without medical supervision.

Throughout his recommendations, Scala mentions the ramifications of common treatments and surgeries for I.B.D. sufferers. He points out, for example, that patients who have had most of their colon removed have lost much of their ability to produce vitamin K and may need to take it in supplemental form.

Finally, Scala addresses the role of stress in terms of I.B.D. flare-ups. He recommends support groups for I.B.D. patients. To have people around who understand the problem, he believes, can lessen much of the emotional stress and consequently reduce the frequency and severity of flare-ups.

NUTRITIONAL EVALUATION The book has neither menus nor formal dietary programs to analyze. The eating guidelines, however, are sound and the foods emphasized should promote a nutritious diet.

PRACTICALITY This book represents a pragmatic approach to inflammatory bowel disease. I.B.D. is an ailment that can often seem beyond the control of the sufferer. By emphasizing those aspects of I.B.D. that *are* within the patient's control, Scala's words can be not only highly useful but soothing and inspiring as well. The style is positive and motivational. Scala attempts to reach out and make a difference in the lives of his readers.

Of particular interest is his advice about monitoring medications. He recommends purchasing *The People's Pharmacy Text* and suggests other ways to investigate important information about the drugs that may be prescribed for I.B.D. and their effects on important nutrients. This effort, while time-consuming, is probably worthwhile: a dedicated interest in health and well-being is especially important for anyone who suffers an incurable illness.

Finally, Scala's advice goes beyond the I.B.D. patient to address those around the patient in the interest of heightened awareness and support.

LIFESTYLE AND EXERCISE Citing emotional stress as an exacerbating factor in I.B.D. flare-ups, Scala offers extensive stress-reduction advice and suggests ways to identify major sources of stress and methods of neutralizing them or converting them into positive energy. He recommends keeping a diary in order to make associations between particular behaviors and I.B.D. flare-ups. He provides specific suggestions for dealing with fatigue and boredom, and he emphasizes that emotional stress is idiosyncratic: one person's stressful situation may be another's calm enjoyment. Above all, he urges the reader to separate that which is controllable from that which is not and to concentrate efforts on the former.

Scala discusses the benefits of physical activity to overall health and its effects on I.B.D. Exercise, for example, helps increase blood circulation, which enhances the body's ability to remove waste. Increased circulation to the brain can also mean less depression due to the release of mood-elevating endorphins. Finally, exercise tones all muscles, including the bowel. Scala recommends starting with vigorous walking for 30 minutes four to five times per week. He includes a good motivational message for why you should start exercising immediately, but he cautions against excessive cycling, swimming, tennis, jogging, or any other activity that can bring on overexertion—a potential cause of I.B.D. flare-ups.

WHY IT WORKS Written in an enjoyable conversational style, this book provides easily managed guidelines to help sufferers of I.B.D. create their own individualized diet for reducing flare-ups and ensuring adequate nutrition. The book has a number of useful charts that illustrate such important information as I.B.D. symptom summaries, food lists, and food preparation methods. All of the advice is tempered with Scala's urging to monitor changes to ensure that food choices, medication, and exercise are appropriate. His advice about supplements is strong—he believes they really make a difference for people with I.B.D.—but he does not go overboard. For example, he discourages the use of amino acid supplements, recommending that these nutrients be obtained from protein food sources instead, to ensure a proper balance.

Scala's advice throughout the book is thorough and well-considered. While he cautions against excess fat and cholesterol, he does not recommend the complete elimination of eggs from the diet. Where extreme measures are called for he recommends them; but where moderation is in order, that is what he advises. This sober approach should be helpful to anyone with I.B.D., a disease that can create a sense of panic. He offers the reader the means to take back control of his or her body to the degree that such control is possible.

POTENTIAL DRAWBACKS   Scala recommends surimi (imitation crab and lobster) for people who cannot eat the real thing without experiencing I.B.D. flare-ups, but he fails to mention that surimi is high in sodium and nutritionally inferior to the foods it replaces. He contradicts himself by listing clams as a food to avoid, then suggesting pasta and clams as an excellent meal. Finally, his statement about the RDA recommendation for vitamin C is incorrect (he says 65 milligrams; it is actually 60), and his mention of eight essential amino acids also just misses (there are really nine).

These are relatively minor point in an otherwise useful, thorough, and accurate piece of work.

SECOND OPINION   "Scala provides straightforward recommendations for healthy eating that's easy on the gut. His writing is frank and concise. . . . Scala knows his subject well and always comes across as hopeful and helpful—without preaching."

—Publishers Weekly

MEDICAL/HEALTH/SPECIALTY DIETS

IRRITABLE BOWEL SYNDROME (I.B.S.)

MORE THAN 30 MILLION Americans suffer from irritable bowel syndrome (I.B.S.), which is characterized by erratic behavior in the muscles of the colon, preventing it from contracting in a coordinated manner, causing spasms that either move food too quickly or too slowly through the gastrointestinal tract. This is a serious dysfunction but should not be confused with I.B.D., which is a *disease* and far more severe.

Many people with I.B.S are unaware that their symptoms are the result of this condition. Those symptoms include severe abdominal pain, alternating attacks of diarrhea and constipation, and the accompanying discomfort and anxiety. For many I.B.S. sufferers, the unpredictability of these symptoms significantly limits activities.

Irritable bowel syndrome is one of the most common digestive disorders and one of the most difficult to treat. There is no definitive diagnostic test or cure. As a result, many people with I.B.S. go from one doctor to another seeking relief, often being misunderstood and misdiagnosed. Others do not seek treatment, either because of fear or embarrassment.

There is help for I.B.S. sufferers. Irritable bowel syndrome can be controlled through a combination of stress management and dietary modifications. The following book, which I co-authored, addresses both of these concerns.

THE WELLNESS BOOK OF I.B.S.: A GUIDE TO LIFELONG RELIEF FROM SYMPTOMS OF ONE OF AMERICA'S MOST COMMON AND LEAST-TALKED-ABOUT AILMENTS: IRRITABLE BOWEL SYNDROME

by Deralee Scanlon, R.D.,
with Barbara Cottman Becnel
St. Martin's Press
New York: 1989

ABOUT THE AUTHORS   My experience as a registered dietitian includes nutritional assessment, diet therapy and counseling, and the special needs related to pregnancy, infancy, the elderly, gastrointestinal disorders, and other specific ailments. I have served as media spokesperson for several companies and associations and have frequently appeared as a nutritional authority on television and radio. I write a weekly column, "Ask The Dietitian," for a number of Southern California newspapers, and my articles on nutrition have appeared in national magazines. I teach nutrition and weight loss classes for Emeritus College and have lectured to organizations on fad dieting, cholesterol reduction, label reading, and nutrition as preventive medicine.

Barbara Cottman Becnel is the author of *The Co-Dependent Parent* and *Parents Who Help Their Children Overcome Drugs*.

OVERVIEW   Since a surprisingly large percentage of people who suffer from I.B.S. know little or nothing about the ailment, the opening chapter of this book is devoted to an explanation of what I.B.S. is—its bodily mechanics, what triggers the symptoms, and how they can be prevented—and what I.B.S. is not. (It is not, for example, a disease.) A detailed discussion differentiates I.B.S. from inflammatory bowel disease (I.B.D.). While the symptoms of I.B.S. can be painful and affect the quality of one's life, it is emphasized that this condition is not considered life-threatening. That fact, once understood, can often relieve a lot of the stress and anxiety that so often brings on the symptoms.

The book also covers the topic of I.B.S. diagnosis, since this illness is so often misdiagnosed or undiagnosed. There remains controversy over the necessity of excessive testing versus minimal testing. Both sides of the argument are presented along with some common techniques of diagnosing the condition, including the thorough patient history interview, known as the LEARN method (L-listen, E-explain, A-acknowledge, R-recommend, N-negotiate agreement for treatment).

Theories on the psychology and physiology of I.B.S. are dealt with along with the three major triggers of I.B.S. symptoms: stress (positive and negative), the effects of certain medications, and reactions to specific foods. Stress-reducing techniques are emphasized, including the following eight:

1. *Biofeedback*, a method in which people are trained to enhance their health by using signals from their own bodies to help reduce tension and anxiety.

2. *Progressive relaxation*, deliberately contracting and releasing major muscle groups.

3. *Differential relaxation*, relaxing through "willing" muscles to let go.

4. *Deep muscle relaxation*, an advanced form combining two and three.

5. *Imagery*, replacing distressing ideas with images and more positive thoughts.

6. *Hypnotherapy*, using a state of heightened suggestibility characterized by increased relaxation and concentration to help control pain and other symptoms.

7. *Laughter*, as a stress breaker.

8. *Exercise*, as a tension reliever and mood elevator.

Along with stress reduction, the book attempts to help the I.B.S. sufferer learn how to prevent I.B.S. symptoms through modifications in daily eating habits. This includes a discussion of food sensitivities and intolerances, which often contribute to symptom attacks, as well as instructions on how to self-test to determine whether you should avoid any specific foods. Several pages are devoted to a chart listing foods that are known to cause problems for many I.B.S. sufferers, along with recommended substitutes.

Readers are shown how to individualize their diet therapy program to manage their symptoms. Suggestions are given about testing for food tolerances. This is called a food challenge; it seeks not only to identify troublesome foods but also to provide a method for easing potentially troublesome foods back into the diet once symptoms have significantly decreased.

The book offers a selection of 50 recipes specially created for I.B.S. comfort, featuring dishes free of those foods most commonly associated with I.B.S. symptoms. These recipes include main dishes, side dishes, soups, breads, and desserts; they are analyzed for their nutritional value, including calories, protein, carbohydrates, and fat. The book also discusses supplements that may aid in digestion and absorption or in healing.

Readers are urged to maintain a "food-mood diary" in order to help them pinpoint the foods, as well as the mealtime conditions, that trigger symptoms. To help overcome those symptoms when they do occur, there is a comprehensive 30-day menu plan covering breakfasts, lunches, dinners, and three daily snacks. Eating six small amounts of food per day, rather than the usual three large meals, can be an effective approach to avoiding I.B.S. and other gastrointestinal discomfort.

Beyond what to eat, the book also provides advice about *how* to eat. Tips are provided for relaxing during mealtimes, eating slowly and chewing thoroughly, and for after-meal walks.

While the book does not promote the use of medications to deal with I.B.S., many physicians find it necessary to prescribe medications for some I.B.S. patients, and so the book describes the most commonly prescribed tranquilizers, as well as common bulking agents, anticholinergics (antispasmodic drugs), and antidiarrheal agents (both narcotic and nonnarcotic).

Throughout the book are case histories of people who are dealing with I.B.S., from moderate discomfort to total homebound debilitation, and who share advice on what has worked for them.

NUTRITIONAL EVALUATION   Averaging two days of the 30-day menu plan, the calories came within the book's recommended 1,800 per day, broken down as follows:

Carbohydrates 59%
Protein 24%
Fat 17%
Sodium . . . . 1,778 milligrams
Fiber . . . . 20 grams
Cholesterol . . . . 433 milligrams

ANALYSIS OF 2-DAY MENU FOR FEMALE, AGE 35

The Wellness Book of I.B.S.

PERCENTAGE OF RA/RM

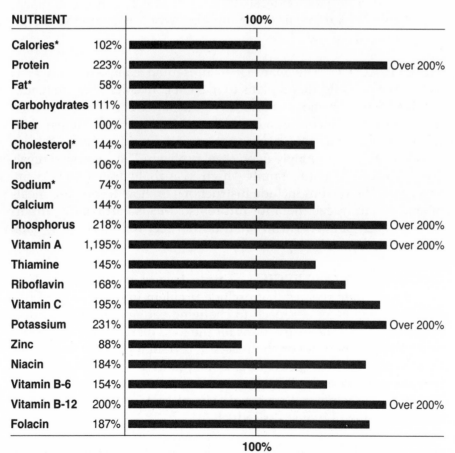

NUTRIENT		100%
Calories*	102%	
Protein	223%	Over 200%
Fat*	58%	
Carbohydrates	111%	
Fiber	100%	
Cholesterol*	144%	
Iron	106%	
Sodium*	74%	
Calcium	144%	
Phosphorus	218%	Over 200%
Vitamin A	1,195%	Over 200%
Thiamine	145%	
Riboflavin	168%	
Vitamin C	195%	
Potassium	231%	Over 200%
Zinc	88%	
Niacin	184%	
Vitamin B-6	154%	
Vitamin B-12	200%	Over 200%
Folacin	187%	

100%

*Recommended maximum allowance. Nutrient should not exceed 100%.

Complex carbohydrates are well within the recommended percentage, but protein is a bit high but acceptable because the carbohydrates and fat levels are within recommended goals. Cholesterol is higher than what is generally recommended. This was largely the result of selecting a particular day's menu that included a whole egg and shrimp. Since most of the 30 days do not contain such high-cholesterol foods, cholesterol should average down to a more advisable level. Also, within a time frame as brief as 30 days, or for use during times of symptom distress, cholesterol should not present a significant health problem. The nutritional objective with I.B.S. is to reduce total fat, especially *saturated* fat, a known cause of symptom attack, and the diet does accomplish this. Fiber and sodium are both within acceptable health goals.

This diet provides at least 100 percent of the RDA for all essential vitamins and minerals except for zinc, which is above the acceptable two-thirds of the RDA.

PRACTICALITY The material is presented complete with lists, charts, recipes, and menu plans to make it convenient for the reader to follow the instructions and dietary guidelines. The stress-reduction techniques are uncomplicated and can be practiced almost anywhere. In general, this book attempts to provide a practical approach to an excruciatingly *im*practical problem. The suggested meals are good for the entire family—high in carbohydrates, low in fat, and tasty. The recipes include instructions on how to prepare meals or snacks and freeze them for future use; this is particularly important for I.B.S. sufferers who often do not feel well enough to cook when symptoms flare up.

LIFESTYLE AND EXERCISE Thirty days of menu plans, along with appropriate recipes that exclude problem foods, give the I.B.S. sufferer a hands-on approach to changing eating behavior to effect positive change. The instructions for the food diary enable the reader to understand how he or she reacts to certain foods and situations. By identifying the triggers of I.B.S. symptoms, the patient can begin to make the necessary dietary and stress-reduction changes.

Exercise, while not essential to treating I.B.S., is addressed as an effective method of stress reduction.

WHY IT WORKS The lists of foods to avoid are accompanied by practical substitutes to help I.B.S. sufferers find those safe comfort foods that are especially important during periods of symptom attack. The diet is, in general, well balanced and includes as much food variety as the individual can tolerate. The menus and recipes are healthful, nutritious, and flavorful, in addition to avoiding those foods most likely to cause I.B.S. flare-ups.

The book educates I.B.S. sufferers in how to manage and gain control of their problem. It provides a therapeutic dietary strategy together with an intensive stress-management program that can put the reader in control of the disorder.

POTENTIAL DRAWBACKS   Although the book's list of foods to avoid during times of distress might be helpful for many I.B.S. sufferers with food intolerances, more caution could have been recommended for pregnant or lactating women. The first week of the 30-day diet plan omits dairy products (in order to test for lactose intolerance) and is thus extremely low in calcium and folacin. On the other hand, one week without adequate calcium or folacin should probably not pose a problem.

In addition, any day of the diet that includes shrimp or a whole egg will be relatively high in cholesterol.

SECOND OPINIONS   "This book is recommended to I.B.S. sufferers who feel left out and confused. . . . The information presented in this book can be used in conjunction with any other treatment prescribed by a physician."

—Current Diet Review

". . . this brief guide provides useful and practical nutritional advice."

—ALA Booklist: The Professional Multimedia Evaluation Service

MEDICAL/HEALTH/SPECIALTY DIETS

LACTOSE INTOLERANCE

LACTOSE INTOLERANCE IS an inability to properly digest lactose, the natural sugar in milk and milk products, due to a lack of the intestinal enzyme lactase. There are three basic types of lactose intolerance:

1. *Congenital*, a rare illness found in newborns.

2. *Primary acquired*, the most common, a genetic disorder that begins early in childhood.

3. *Secondary acquired*, resulting from a disease, most commonly a viral intestinal infection but also other illnesses such as celiac or Crohn's disease, intestinal parasites such as Giardia, from medication such as antibiotics and cancer drugs, or from surgery such as ulcer operations or bowel resection.

Lactose intolerance affects approximately 60 million people in North America alone, including between 70 percent and 90 percent of all people of African and Asian descent, and is the most common cause of diarrhea and/or gaseousness. Other symptoms include (in varying degrees) stomach rumbling, bloating, flatulence, and cramping.

The following book presents an approach to avoiding those symptoms through lactose-free eating.

THE MILK SUGAR DILEMMA: LIVING WITH LACTOSE INTOLERANCE

by Richard A. Martens, M.D. and
Sherlyn Martens, M.S., R.D.
Medi-Ed Press
East Lansing, Michigan: 1987

ABOUT THE AUTHORS   Dr. Martens is a clinical gastroenterologist educated at DePaul, Bradley, and the University of Illinois College of Medicine. He received a fellowship in gastroenterology at Yale, and his medical school teaching appointments include the University of Illinois, Northwestern, and Loyola University. Since 1970 he has maintained a private practice in consultative gastroenterology.

Sherlyn Martens is a clinical registered dietitian. A graduate of Michigan State University, she is in private practice for the Gastroenterology Association of East Lansing, Michigan.

OVERVIEW   The goal of this book is to give a clear, nonmedical description of the condition and to provide a program of dietary management. The authors offer a detailed description of lactose intolerance, including a diagram comparing proper digestive absorption and lactose intolerance. They advance an evolutionary theory of why this allergy is so common in human beings: that in order to discourage older children from returning to the breast when younger children have to be nursed, the older children develop an intolerance to milk sugar.

The authors then discuss diagnosis, reviewing the usual tests and observatory practices and giving their recommendations, including do-it-yourself tests that can save the patient money without necessarily compromising accuracy. According to the authors, lactose intolerance differs in degree from one individual to another. They describe how to establish your own tolerance level.

In their program for lactose-restricted eating, the authors emphasize the replacement of milk's nutrients, primarily calcium, vitamin D, vitamin A, and riboflavin, to ensure adequate nutrition with or without vitamin and mineral supplementation. Nutritional guidelines are given, including a breakdown of USRDA calcium requirements for children, adults, premenopausal and postmenopausal women, and pregnant and lactating women. The authors discuss the perils of osteoporosis and the role of calcium and vitamin D in helping to prevent it. The book offers a lactose-restricted menu planner with a wide variety of foods. This planner breaks lactose-restricted foods into the three basic groups—protein, carbohydrate, and fat. It highlights those foods high in the nutrients found otherwise in milk and milk products. The plan provides sample menus but is also designed to allow the dieter to make his or her own selections. It includes special considerations for vegetarians, who run nutrient deficiency risks when avoiding milk products, especially in terms of protein, iron, zinc, calcium, riboflavin, and vitamins D and B-12.

The authors also devote attention to various milk substitutes, comparing taste, use, and calories. Since aging reduces the lactose content in many cheeses, the authors provide a list of aging times in cheeses and their resulting lactose levels.

Other tips include approaches to dining out and parties. Since lactose-intolerance management depends upon making informed decisions, the authors include a self-quiz to reinforce the reader's awareness and ability to spot lactose-containing foods.

NUTRITIONAL EVALUATION   Since the diet does not specify portion size, I used standard portion sizes for analysis. Given that, the caloric level was reasonable and the breakdown of the major nutrients was as follows:

Carbohydrates	47%
Protein	21%
Fat	32%
Sodium	1,722 milligrams
Fiber	15 grams
Cholesterol	159 milligrams

Protein and fat are slightly above recommended goals while carbohydrates are below the suggested minimum. Probably because of this ratio, fiber is lower than what is required to promote good health. On the positive side, sodium and cholesterol are well within recommended goals.

All essential micronutrients meet 100 percent of the RDA guidelines except for iron, thiamine, riboflavin, potassium, zinc, and niacin, which all meet at least two-thirds of the RDA (zinc, in fact, is at 96 percent).

An increase in complex carbohydrates, especially fruits and whole-grain products, should not only improve the carbohydrate/protein/fat ratio but also bolster the intake of niacin, thiamine, riboflavin, iron, and potassium, in addition to fiber.

ANALYSIS OF 1-DAY MENU FOR FEMALE, AGE 35

The Milk Sugar Dilemma

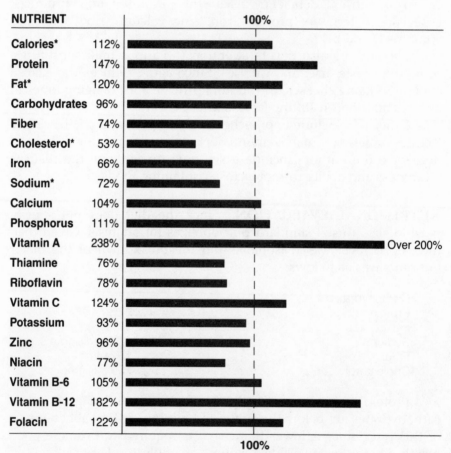

PERCENTAGE OF RA/RM

NUTRIENT		100%
Calories*	112%	
Protein	147%	
Fat*	120%	
Carbohydrates	96%	
Fiber	74%	
Cholesterol*	53%	
Iron	66%	
Sodium*	72%	
Calcium	104%	
Phosphorus	111%	
Vitamin A	238%	Over 200%
Thiamine	76%	
Riboflavin	78%	
Vitamin C	124%	
Potassium	93%	
Zinc	96%	
Niacin	77%	
Vitamin B-6	105%	
Vitamin B-12	182%	
Folacin	122%	

100%

*Recommended maximum allowance. Nutrient should not exceed 100%.

PRACTICALITY The narrative is easy reading and the information is well researched. No one ever said food intolerances were a convenient condition, and avoiding lactose may not always be pleasant. But this program can make it a lot easier with extensive lists of manufacturers and their lactose-free food products, including a list of milk substitutes such as Lactaid, an enzyme-treated milk, and enzyme drops that can be added to milk. *The Milk Sugar Dilemma* offers useful tips for eating out, parties, and vacations. The authors recommend lactase pills, which will help in the digestion of lactose when a dining situation necessitates consuming milk products. They warn about Chinese restaurants, which often mix monosodium glutamate (MSG), with lactose powder to promote thickening and rapid dissolving.

Additionally, the authors offer tips on selecting low-lactose fast foods, school lunches, typical office party fare, and even nursing home foods—everything from appetizers to desserts. They suggest how to avoid embarrassment in social gatherings despite having to adhere to a modified diet.

LIFESTYLE AND EXERCISE The book itself is a behavioral modification tool, reassuring readers by letting them know how common this problem is and by describing the least intrusive way to live with it. The self-quiz is not only a learning tool but a good attitude boost. Identifying and avoiding lactose can be approached as an annoying chore or as a challenge.

Exercise is not addressed in this book, perhaps under the assumption that it has no direct effect on lactose intolerance.

WHY IT WORKS *The Milk Sugar Dilemma* is a clear and concise layperson's approach to lactose intolerance. It gives the reader access not only to food intolerance management but also to some facts about the condition. Some data that are usually reserved for medical journals are presented here in understandable terms. The book demystifies the condition and may make it seem less daunting.

The eating plan stresses a variety of lactose-free and lactose-restricted foods to ensure adequate overall nutrition and foster general health. The book sets out to create educated consumers. The useful information about label reading, nutrient replacement, vegetarianism, shopping, and eating out promotes independent coping skills that can last a lifetime.

POTENTIAL DRAWBACKS Though well-researched, the book includes some minor erroneous statements—for example, that airlines may require a physician's order as a prerequisite to furnishing a lactose-free meal. Most airlines are very cooperative in accommodating the dietary needs of passengers; although they generally do not have a special meal called "lactose free," if you explain that you need a "milk free" meal, they can usually provide one.

Also, this book does not always consider overall health as being as important as managing lactose intolerance. One example is in the advice for ordering from a limited restaurant breakfast menu: the authors' recommendations include butter, bacon, ham, and eggs. These all contribute to high fat intake and the health problems that go with it. Such recommendations are not in keeping with the balanced menus provided in the book.

SECOND OPINION "This is a well-organized text providing complete and practical information for lactose-intolerant individuals."

—*Journal of the American Dietetic Association*

MEDICAL/HEALTH/SPECIALTY DIETS

MULTIPLE SCLEROSIS (MS)

MS, AS IT IS COMMONLY known, is a chronic and progressive disease of the central nervous system in which the protective layer surrounding the brain and nerve tissue is damaged. This causes random multiple lesions in the brain and spinal cord, interfering with or blocking nerve impulses throughout the body and impeding proper body functioning.

According to clinical observations and available objective data, the incidence of MS has increased during this century. It is, in fact, considered to be a modern disease; few, if any, cases were known before the nineteenth century. One theory is that a diet high in animal fat—common only in recent history—is largely responsible for the onset of MS.

Multiple sclerosis is considered a disease of young adults; 85 percent of MS patients experience their first symptoms between ages 20 and 35. Before becoming disabled, the typical person who will be afflicted with MS is active, energetic, highly productive, of average height and weight, athletic, attractive, perceptive, and on the nervous side. Interestingly, because they usually fit this personality type, most MS sufferers whose symptoms do not severely disable them maintain their desire to work, generally become well-informed about their disease, and are aggressive in coping with it. Risk for MS is believed to have a genetic component, which may be latent for two or three generations. The disease is also believed to affect equal numbers of men and women, although it seems to affect men more severely. This may be because men do not seek treatment for their symptoms as readily as do women.

These symptoms can include nervous tension, irritability, fatigue, a low tolerance for emotional or psychological stress, memory impairment (especially regarding recent events), cold feet and hands, feeling cold despite being in a warm room, hot spells, night sweats, and bruising easily.

Most people with MS have low blood pressure and a slightly elevated (though not abnormally so) blood-sugar level. Male sufferers may experience partial or total loss of sexual potency, while females may have loss of sex drive. Other symptoms of MS may include scintillating scotoma (focal impaired vision), sometimes associated with migraine headaches, nausea, and vomiting. They also have a low tolerance for heat or for any temperature change of more than 20 degrees Fahrenheit, as well as an intolerance for alcohol, suffering severe hangovers from even a small intake of alcohol.

Dietary measures, if started when MS symptoms first appear, have been found to influence the effects of the disease and keep it in remission, allowing a productive and high-quality life. Once the disease has progressed, dietary modifications can no longer lead to remission but can still slow the degenerative process. The following book addresses how changes in diet can make a difference for multiple sclerosis patients.

THE MULTIPLE SCLEROSIS DIET BOOK: A LOW-FAT DIET FOR THE TREATMENT OF MS

by Roy Laver Swank, M.D., Ph.D.,
and Barbara Brewer Dugan
Doubleday
New York: 1987

ABOUT THE AUTHORS Dr. Swank is a graduate of Northwestern University Medical School. He has previously published *The Swank Low-Fat Diet*, of which this is an extensive revision. He has devoted 36 years to investigating multiple sclerosis and has authored numerous scientific papers on the subject. He owns the patents on a number of MS-related medical inventions. Swank has received several awards for research and is listed in *Who's Who in Science, Who's Who in America,* and *Who's Who in the World.* He is currently Professor Emeritus of Neurology at Oregon Health Sciences University.

Barbara Brewer Dugan is a research associate in the Department of Neurology at Oregon Health Sciences University.

OVERVIEW This book sets out to give multiple sclerosis sufferers a more complete understanding of their disease—its history, possible causes, and therapeutic options—so that they can achieve the maximum benefits by beginning effective treatment immediately. Major research findings are summarized, including Swank's own, which found that saturated fat causes clumping of red blood cells in laboratory animals very much like the clumping of blood found in MS patients.

Swank's theory about saturated fat and MS does not stop there. He presents a correlation between countries with typical diets high in saturated fats and their high incidence of multiple sclerosis. His dietary recommendations are very low in saturated fat. Over the past 20 years, this diet has resulted in a positive correlation between the reduction in saturated fat and a decrease in deterioration and death among MS patients.

Swank discusses the importance of early diagnosis; the earlier dietary and other measures are taken, the more profound the results. He points out that MS is not reversible, but that its

251

progression can be halted through modifications in diet and life-style. The author explains how the symptoms unfold, emphasizing the early signs, of which persistent fatigue is most common. He also discusses the methods by which doctors make clinical diagnoses of MS.

According to Swank, the best response to a diagnosis of MS at *any* stage begins with a diet very low in saturated fat. He advises a fat intake of less than four teaspoons of saturated fat per day (20 grams)—as little as three teaspoons (15 grams), if possible. In Swank's research, even those who ate *five* teaspoons had an increased death rate. Swank also recommends consuming 20 to 50 grams of *polyunsaturated* oil per day.

He discusses the major food groups and nutrients as they relate to MS, then makes these eight specific dietary recommendations:

1. No red meat or dark-meat poultry for the first year.

2. After the first year, three ounces of red meat or dark-meat poultry per week.

3. Nonfat dairy products only, except for one serving (one cup milk or one ounce cheese) of 1 percent dairy products per day.

4. No processed foods containing saturated fat.

5. Saturated fat *never* to exceed 15 grams (three teaspoons) per day.

6. A minimum of four teaspoons (20 grams) per day of polyunsaturated vegetable oils—as much as 10 teaspoons (50 grams) per day.

7. One teaspoon (or four capsules) of nonconcentrated cod-liver oil and one multiple vitamin/mineral tablet per day.

8. Recording all fat consumption, measuring fats/oils in teaspoons.

Swank also lists permissible and forbidden foods and offers specific advice for MS patients who need to lose or gain weight and for particularly active people. The book contains over 350 recipes, including meatless meals, desserts, muffins and breads, vegetable side dishes, sauces, soups, meat and seafood dishes, and ethnic cuisine, along with one week of sample menus. Specific examples show how to distribute fats and oils throughout the day. Swank also includes tips for eating out, traveling, and cooking.

In directly treating MS patients, Swank has them keep food diaries to be evaluated by a registered dietitian while their physical condition is checked by a physician. But the emphasis is always on patient self-care.

Swank's advice goes beyond diet. He points out that alcohol, caffeine, tobacco, and marijuana can promote and aggravate MS symptom attacks. According to Swank, multiple sclerosis is also made worse by anxiety, fatigue, irritability, and depression; he answers each of these problems with advice on stress reduction, dealing with personal crisis, and relaxation. He advises, for example, a one- to two-hour midday nap as part of MS therapy to prevent fatigue. Perhaps most important, he gives advice on how to assume a positive attitude about living with the limitations of the disease.

NUTRITIONAL EVALUATION Analyzing one of the seven days of sample menus, I find the calories higher than the book recommends, but still within an acceptable range. They break down as follows:

```
Carbohydrates ........................... 48%
Protein ..................................... 20%
Fat ......................................... 32%
Sodium ..................................... 1,283 milligrams
Fiber ....................................... 19 grams
Cholesterol ............................... 167 milligrams
```

Protein is within the pre-1989 RDA goals, which I would consider satisfactory, but carbohydrates are low even by those standards, and fat is above the acceptable maximum—due in part to the author's recommending 50 grams of polyunsaturated fat per day. Dieters should probably adjust for this by lowering other dietary fat. Cholesterol is well within established goals, reflecting the emphasis on low saturated fat consumption. Fiber is slightly below the recommended range, but the author does suggest the use of whole-grain products to increase fiber.

All essential vitamins and minerals meet 100 percent of the RDA guidelines except for zinc, which is above two-thirds of those guidelines, and iron, which is not. Since red meat is restricted for

ANALYSIS OF 1-DAY MENU FOR FEMALE, AGE 35

The Multiple Sclerosis Diet

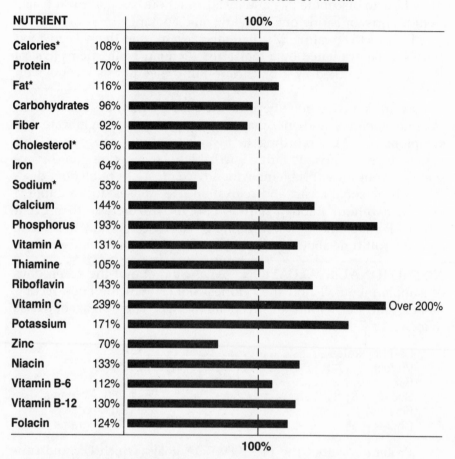

PERCENTAGE OF RA/RM

NUTRIENT		
Calories*	108%	
Protein	170%	
Fat*	116%	
Carbohydrates	96%	
Fiber	92%	
Cholesterol*	56%	
Iron	64%	
Sodium*	53%	
Calcium	144%	
Phosphorus	193%	
Vitamin A	131%	
Thiamine	105%	
Riboflavin	143%	
Vitamin C	239%	Over 200%
Potassium	171%	
Zinc	70%	
Niacin	133%	
Vitamin B-6	112%	
Vitamin B-12	130%	
Folacin	124%	

100%

*Recommended maximum allowance. Nutrient should not exceed 100%.

the first year on this diet, the best food sources of iron would be whole grains, enriched cereals, and dried beans and peas. The use of lemon juice and other vitamin C sources can aid in iron absorption.

PRACTICALITY Avoiding saturated fat is not always easy, but Swank's method is about as simple, straightforward, and sensible as can be expected. The necessity of reading food labels will make grocery trips take longer, and the need to avoid hydrogenated oils may create shopping frustrations and send you reeling to the nearest health food store. But, like anything else, frequent experience at label reading can make you an expert and considerably decrease the annoyance and time. Besides, feeling better is worth any effort.

Swank advises dining out only once a week, which may be impractical for some, but his tips can help those who cannot adhere to this restriction to do as much as possible to control the amount of saturated fat they consume in restaurant meals. These tips include effective ways of communicating your dietary needs to a waiter and what to do when in doubt (for example, do not eat the salad dressing if you cannot get a positive identification of the oil in it).

The tips for eating while traveling include suggestions for breakfasts, lunches, and dinners in terms of the type of restaurant to look for and what to order. On the subject of traveling abroad, Swank recommends avoiding "Bed & Breakfast" inns in favor of hotels with restaurants that provide greater variety. With regard to vacations in general, he suggests stretching your saturated fat limit up to 20 grams per day to allow for greater flexibility (provided the vacation does not exceed three weeks).

Swank's cooking advice addresses the specific problems of the disabled MS sufferer, as well as methods of ensuring low fat, including tips on how to convert favorite recipes. The tables of permissible foods and their quantities should help not only in meal preparation but in record keeping. The use of a food scale may be an annoyance for some, but should only be necessary for certain fatty fishes.

As for his cod-liver oil recommendations, Swank does acknowledge its fishy taste and suggests a fruit juice chaser as well as the use of cod-liver oil capsules when traveling.

No special foods are required, and the dietary restrictions should promote overall health for the MS patient and for anyone else. Most of these guidelines can be applied uniformly to the whole family.

Along with being thorough, the book is clear and well organized, although it would have helped if the recipe page numbers were listed on the menus for convenient reference.

LIFESTYLE AND EXERCISE Swank pays particular attention to the behavioral aspects of MS and its treatment. His suggested food diary can help in the adoption of a new eating regimen, and his recommendations on stress management, fatigue prevention, and a positive attitude are well presented. The theme of the book seems to be: You can contain and control MS by doing things that are completely within your power.

Exercise is not discussed as a part of treatment. Swank does caution MS patients who wish to exercise to avoid becoming fatigued.

WHY IT WORKS With thirty-six years of research behind him, Swank is clearly one of the foremost authorities on multiple sclerosis. His program is based upon firsthand experience as a doctor and researcher, and the theories upon which his diet are based have been well documented and accepted by others in the field.

The Multiple Sclerosis Diet Book's program, which is used in clinics throughout the United States, provides step-by-step advice on how to utilize the data in order to stop the degeneration of MS. Swank makes the reader a knowledgeable MS patient and then describes how to put that knowledge to work.

POTENTIAL DRAWBACKS This diet demands considerable self-discipline, ingenuity, and, at the very least, a major adjustment period that can last for several months—during which time fatigue and irritability may get worse before they get better. This, however, is a small price to pay in order to halt MS in its tracks. Also, while most of the charts are clear and helpful, some may be confusing to the average reader. Finally, as in several other diet books, clams, scallops, and oysters are grouped together with shrimp, crab, and lobster, although the former are considerably lower in cholesterol.

SECOND OPINION ". . . the fact that 95 percent of the dieters have remained well and active for over 30 years strongly suggests that an unsaturated fat diet can be helpful in controlling this normally progressive disease."

—Health Gazette

MEDICAL/HEALTH/SPECIALTY DIETS

POST-CORONARY

IT IS NO SECRET THAT HEART disease and heart attacks have a strong link to dietary habits, but there is much confusion among the general public about which dietary habits need to be changed and how to improve them.

A heart attack is survivable; many people not only recover but achieve a level of health and well-being far beyond what they had thought possible. But such transformation is possible only through information and education. Although some doctors are better than others at providing patients with that awareness, you do not need to rely on your physician alone. The following book can enhance your knowledge in this area.

An Affair of the Heart
(A Heart-to-Heart Guide
for Post-Coronary Care)

by Phyllis Denny
Ashley Books, Inc.
Port Washington, NY: 1988

ABOUT THE AUTHOR A self-described renaissance woman, Denny is a motion picture producer, director, and writer as well as an author of short stories and books. Two of her films were medical documentaries, one on heart disease, the other on stress. Both received the John Muir Medical Film Festival Award. Denny has first-hand knowledge of this subject; she helped her husband recover from a severe heart attack after departing the hospital with no more than this medical advice: "Keep him quiet, give him a low-sodium, low-cholesterol diet, monitor his medication, and see me in two weeks."

OVERVIEW This book's plan is much more than a diet. It is a comprehensive program to help heart attack survivors and those who care for them through what can be a traumatic period but can also be the beginning of a healthier and better way of life. Denny's advice, while often focusing on nutrition, pays close attention to the logistical and, most important, the emotional realities of the situation.

The program begins with a brief education in some of the physiological realities of heart disease: the causes of heart attacks and ways to prevent their occurrence and recurrence. Next, the author applies information about sodium and cholesterol control to the real-world tasks of shopping and meal preparation. She describes ways to serve low-sodium, low-fat, low-cholesterol meals and snacks without sacrificing all of the flavor and enjoyment. The emphasis is on a "healthful gourmet" approach, including tips for using herbs and nonsalty spices to enhance taste.

Along with describing what to eat, the program also lists foods to avoid—some obvious, some not so obvious. It recommends ways to obtain complete and balanced nutrition within the post-coronary food restrictions to assure maximum recovery and prevent other illness.

Heart disease is a many-faceted illness, and this program is appropriately many-faceted. Denny prepares the reader for a number of potential emotional and logistical pitfalls and then provides approaches to sidestep them. She describes, for example, some physical and emotional stresses—those caused by restlessness and boredom, by financial worry and other pressures—and shares her personal history of coping with them.

Denny furnishes a timetable to give the reader an approximate idea of what to expect in terms of recuperation and resuming activities. She also gives instructions on monitoring recovery between doctor visits, to enable you to be a full participant in you recovery.

This plan has no specific food program—that remains the domain of the supervising physician—but it does fill in some potentially wide gaps in the doctor's typical advice to a coronary patient. The recommendations emphasize a diet not only low in sodium, fat, and cholesterol, but also in refined sugar—an important factor in overall health that can help enhance recovery from a heart attack.

NUTRITIONAL EVALUATION Since the book gives no structured diet plan, I analyzed a sample day's menus (provided by a vice president of Ashley Books) based upon the book's various recipes. Since the menu contained no portion sizes, I used standard ones. Thus, while the calories were within a good range, they could vary significantly between individuals. Those calories break down as follows:

Carbohydrates	35%
Protein	43%
Fat	22%
Sodium	374 milligrams
Fiber	8 grams
Cholesterol	220 milligrams

Fat, cholesterol, and sodium, all very important to cardiovascular health, are well within nationally recommended goals. Carbohydrates and fiber, however, are significantly low, and protein is double the pre-1989 U.S. dietary goals that were current when this book was written. I would suggest the following modifications: larger servings from whole-grains, breads, cereals, vegetables, and other complex carbohydrates, and reduced protein portions.

Of the essential micronutrients, only vitamin B-6, vitamin C, niacin, and potassium meet or exceed 100 percent of the RDA.

ANALYSIS OF 1-DAY MENU FOR MALE, AGE 35

An Affair of the Heart

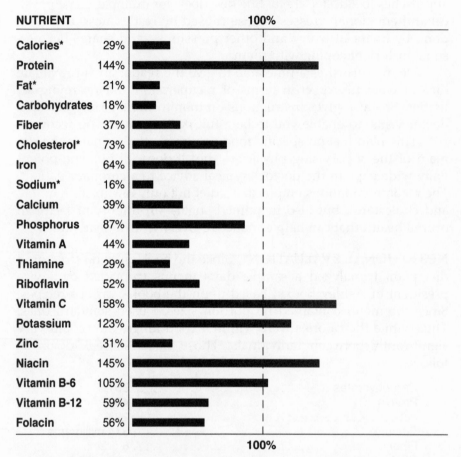

PERCENTAGE OF RA/RM

NUTRIENT		100%
Calories*	29%	
Protein	144%	
Fat*	21%	
Carbohydrates	18%	
Fiber	37%	
Cholesterol*	73%	
Iron	64%	
Sodium*	16%	
Calcium	39%	
Phosphorus	87%	
Vitamin A	44%	
Thiamine	29%	
Riboflavin	52%	
Vitamin C	158%	
Potassium	123%	
Zinc	31%	
Niacin	145%	
Vitamin B-6	105%	
Vitamin B-12	59%	
Folacin	56%	

100%

*Recommended maximum allowance. Nutrient should not exceed 100%.

Phosphorus is above two-thirds of the RDA. The other nutrients are low. Increasing whole-grains, enriched cereals, beans, peas, and dark leafy vegetables will improve most of these nutrient levels. If consuming sufficient amounts of food is a problem for the post-coronary patient, a multiple vitamin/mineral supplement not exceeding 100% of the RDA may provide added insurance. To be on the safe side, check with your physician before starting any supplementation program.

PRACTICALITY   Practicality may be the most appealing element of the book; its objective is to help the post-coronary patient adapt to a potentially difficult lifestyle alteration. The advice is pragmatic and accessible, based primarily on personal experience. The author even provides healthful suggestions for the creative use of leftovers. The nutritional advice can be applied to the entire family—and, in many cases, *should* be.

LIFESTYLE AND EXERCISE   The author recognizes the necessity of modifying behavior along with diet. She recommends record-keeping for self-awareness and a sense of progress. She also suggests uniformly healthful meals for the entire family to prevent the feeling that the heart patient's meals are some sort of special medicine.

As for the emotional effects of post-coronary recovery, Denny lends her own words of encouragement and urges open communication about fears and other negative emotions. She also broaches the subject of professional counseling, encouraging the reader not to be afraid to seek such assistance.

The author recognizes the eventual need for an exercise program, and encourages light exercise as soon as medical approval is given, but she makes no specific recommendations.

WHY IT WORKS   This program stresses variety and moderation, two important elements of good health and well-being that are especially important to post-coronary patients, who may wonder anxiously if they have permanently lost the pleasures of life. The recipe section contains approximately 75 entries and is generous and imaginative, including menus for all occasions. The program also provides the means for creating healthful versions of favorite *un*healthful recipes. The book is written in a humorous and upbeat style for easy, fast, and enjoyable reading.

POTENTIAL DRAWBACKS   Some of the nutritional advice is a bit unsound; for example, the author suggests cutting down on bread— a complex carbohydrate that is relatively low in calories—and recommends cooking vegetables in water for 20 to 30 minutes, a practice that is sure to leach out many nutrients. Light steaming is much better. She also advises the use of polyunsaturated instead of monounsaturated oils. Recent evidence suggests that monounsaturated oils are healthier in terms of cholesterol reduction, which should be a priority for anyone recovering from a heart attack.

The recipes are not accompanied by any nutritional breakdown, and thus I would recommend this book be used along with a basic nutrition book that includes food tables.

SECOND OPINION   "Everything you read has been 'patient-tested.' Over the past ten years, Phyllis has put each and every one of the precepts into living operation. She started by translating her understanding of her husband into principles that work."

—*Moss David Posner, M.D.,*
Internist, San Clemente, California

MEDICAL/HEALTH/SPECIALTY DIETS

WHEAT INTOLERANCE

THIS IS AN AILMENT WITH many names: ce-
liac sprue, celiac disease, adult celiac disease, idiopathic steatorrhea,
nontropical sprue, and gluten-induced enteropathy. It has come to
be known most commonly as gluten intolerance, a term that is
scientifically inaccurate. Wheat contains two proteins; gluten and
gliadin. It is *gliadin* that many people cannot tolerate; however, since
wheat contains both proteins, avoiding one means avoiding the
other—so the inaccuracy is not a perilous one.

By whatever name, this is a common nutritional sensitivity. It is
estimated that as many as 130,000 Americans are intolerant to gliadin. People with this problem vary in degree of sensitivity; some
can consume more wheat than others without suffering the symptoms of bloating, gas pain, diarrhea or constipation, open lesions or
blisters in the gastrointestinal tract, weight loss, anemia, and malnutrition (the last three a consequence of malabsorption of vital
nutrients caused by damage to the surface of the small intestine).

Since the 1960s, the standard treatment for this illness, as with
most common food intolerances, has been to avoid the food you can
not tolerate. This, of course, is easier for someone allergic to radishes
than for someone intolerant to wheat and wheat products. Gluten-
free eating is a challenge that should not be taken on without the
ammunition of good nutritional resources. The following book can
be a good start in building such an arsenal.

THE GLUTEN FREE GOURMET (LIVING WELL WITHOUT WHEAT)

by Betty Hagman
Henry Holt and Company, Inc.
New York: 1990

ABOUT THE AUTHOR   Betty Hagman is a writer and a founding member of the Gluten Intolerance Group (GIG) of North America. Since being diagnosed with celiac sprue (the illness commonly known as gluten intolerance), she has spent 15 years developing recipes to add variety to what could otherwise be a boring diet. Hagman has experimented extensively with nonwheat flours and has developed over 200 recipes, many of which she shares in this book.

OVERVIEW   The book begins with a kind of self-defense manual for people with gluten intolerance, describing hidden sources of gluten in common foods, food products, and restaurant dishes. This includes a lesson on reading food labels, with an enumeration of some key gluten clues such as "modified food starch" as well as some key distinctions; for example, how to tell if distilled vinegar contains gluten and which food additives should be avoided. Hagman details some nonfood gluten sources as well, such as the fillers in tablet and capsule medicines and the glue in some envelope flaps.

Next the author discusses the use of various alternative flours, and ways to overcome their limitations in creating a moist and springy baked product. She also discusses wheat alternatives in nonbaked foods such as meat dishes and salad dressings.

Extensive lists differentiate the many acceptable foods from unacceptable ones, a kind of vocabulary study guide for the wheat intolerant. There are survival tips for dining out, parties, and travel. As an added bonus, dairy substitutes are included for those who are both gluten *and* lactose intolerant.

This diet has no progression or long-range goal. Its purpose is simply to help readers begin immediately to cultivate a diet devoid of gluten and yet high in variety and enjoyment.

NUTRITIONAL EVALUATION With no formal menu plans, I selected from the book's typical breakfasts, lunches, and dinners, using standard portion sizes, since none were provided. My analysis found calories within an acceptable range; remember that this assumes moderate portion size.

Carbohydrates 63%
Protein 13%
Fat 24%
Sodium . . . . 2,664 milligrams
Fiber . . . . 10 grams
Cholesterol . . . . 269 milligrams

Protein, carbohydrate, fat, and cholesterol are all within recommended goals. Sodium, however, is too high, though the author does present ways to use herbs and spices to cut sodium. Fiber is low—though, again, the author offers advice on boosting the fiber numbers by using brown rice flour along with high-fiber vegetables.

All essential micronutrients meet or exceed 100 percent of the RDA except for Vitamin B-6, iron, thiamine, and niacin, which exceed two-thirds of the RDA, and zinc, which does not.

PRACTICALITY Some of the author's suggestions may not be practical for everyone. Cooking from scratch, for example, may be the best way to control ingredients, but it is time consuming and, for some people, impossible. Several of the alternative flours are more readily available than others, and though the author provides helpful advice on where to find them, she also recommends buying a flour mill to process flours yourself. This may be fun and adventurous for some but is likely to be time-consuming and annoying for others. For those who do have the time for home flour processing and baking, these recipes render foods that are not only gluten free but also taste good enough to serve to the entire family.

The author's advice in dealing with restaurants, party hosts, and others responsible for food preparation implies a great degree of trust in these people, which may or may not be appropriate. You may insist that your hash browns not be cooked in oil that has been used to fry pancakes, but good luck enforcing your request. (Of course, many restaurants are cooperative, and so are many friends and party hosts.) Given the realities of life, the author's suggestions

ANALYSIS OF 1-DAY MENU FOR FEMALE, AGE 35

The Gluten Free Gourmet

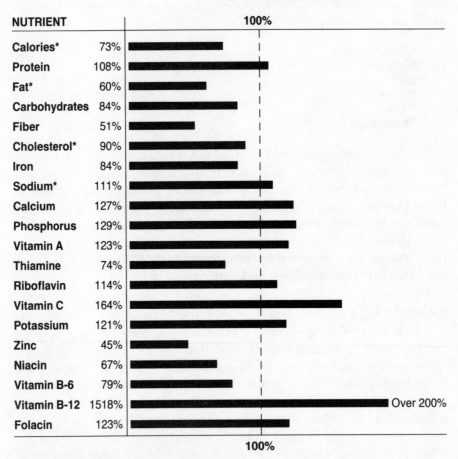

PERCENTAGE OF RA/RM

NUTRIENT		
Calories*	73%	
Protein	108%	
Fat*	60%	
Carbohydrates	84%	
Fiber	51%	
Cholesterol*	90%	
Iron	84%	
Sodium*	111%	
Calcium	127%	
Phosphorus	129%	
Vitamin A	123%	
Thiamine	74%	
Riboflavin	114%	
Vitamin C	164%	
Potassium	121%	
Zinc	45%	
Niacin	67%	
Vitamin B-6	79%	
Vitamin B-12	1518%	Over 200%
Folacin	123%	

100%

*Recommended maximum allowance. Nutrient should not exceed 100%.

for dining out, travel, parties, and holidays probably represent the right approach. They can be the beginning of a successful adaptation and compromise.

LIFESTYLE AND EXERCISE   Lifestyle is not stressed as a particular challenge. The symptoms that result from eating wheat are probably enough of an incentive to ensure a continuing desire to avoid it, and the insights in this book should help make the job easier.

The author does not discuss exercise as an issue related to wheat intolerance. Since physical activity presumably doesn't have much impact on this illness, the omission makes sense, though dieters (and everyone else) should be urged to exercise in the interest of general health and well-being.

WHY IT WORKS The book is a wealth of information for anyone with a wheat intolerance. The approach is simple: avoid the offending substance. The alternatives are presented as being satisfying enough to make this intolerance tolerable. It is a real hands-on approach, with lists not only of what to eat but of where to get it. The book also suggests further modifications for people who need to avoid other foods (sugar, dairy products, and cholesterol) and suggests ways to increase fiber from nonwheat sources.

The author urges readers not to allow complacency—a gluten intolerant's worst enemy—to cause them to eat carelessly and risk suffering the symptoms.

POTENTIAL DRAWBACKS Although the recipes in this book are devoid of wheat products, a number of them do not adhere to all other criteria for health. Some recipes are high in calories, cholesterol, and sodium. Thus, anyone concerned with overall health may need to supplement the advice in this book with that in a more general nutrition book.

SECOND OPINION "Her recipes use flours other than wheat flour, but they are generally uncomplicated and quick to prepare— suitable even for those non-cooks who have been craving their forbidden foods. There are few other cookbooks in this area."

—*Library Journal*

MEDICAL/HEALTH/SPECIALTY DIETS

CONSULTING A REGISTERED DIETITIAN

EFFECTIVE DIET PROGRAMS provide varying degrees of personal attention. As I have pointed out, very low calorie diet programs are designed to be administered under medical and other supervision. Enrollment programs do this to a lesser degree. Yet even those programs which offer the most personal attention may not offer the ongoing involvement of a personal dietitian. For this reason—be it to control weight or to manage a medical condition—it is worth exploring the option of consulting a registered dietitian in order to ensure the maximum degree of individualized care to meet your specific needs and objectives.

In the field of nutrition, as it relates to health and weight management, registered dietitians are, as a profession, widely regarded for their expertise. It is estimated that there are 50,000 or more RDs currently practicing in the United States, providing many different services. Some are responsible for planning the meals served in schools, hospitals, and other institutions while others hold positions in the food manufacturing and retailing industries. Perhaps the greatest number of registered dietitians offer their services to clients on a consulting basis, either individually or in small groups.

Registered dietitians in private practice can provide diet and nutrition information, create an individualized diet regimen for you, or work with you in conjunction with any effective diet plan—such as those recommended in these pages—helping you adapt it to your own particular objectives and personal lifestyle requirements. Regular visits with a personal RD can track your progress and afford the opportunity to make adjustments as needed.

One significant benefit often associated with consulting a registered dietitian is the attention paid to the behavioral modification aspects of diet. RDs can also provide nutrition education, tips on healthier food preparation techniques, recipe modification, advice about exercise, and food label reading.

For medical conditions in which diet plays a substantial role in treatment—such as diabetes and heart disease—an RD can consult and work in tandem with a client's personal physician to ensure that all dietary modifications will be safe and effective. Indeed, some RDs maintain their private practices in association with one or more physicians, psychologists, or exercise physiologists.

A registered dietitian is someone with a Bachelor of Science degree from a college with a specific broad-based course curriculum accredited by the American Dietetic Association (ADA). Upon graduation, an RD candidate must intern for a full year in hospitals and/or clinics. He or she must then successfully pass an all-day written examination (similar in concept to an attorney's Bar exam).

Every state in the U.S. has its own chapter of the American Dietetic Association, and a listing of member RDs is often available. You can obtain the address of the chapter in your area by contacting the national headquarters of the ADA at:

216 West Jackson Blvd, Suite 800
Chicago, Illinois 60606-6995
(312) 899-0040

You can also consult your telephone directory for the names of local registered dietitians. Consultation fees can vary widely. A realistic range is between $40 and $125 per hour; in some cases, Medicare and some medical insurance policies will pay part of the cost.

If you decide to consult a registered dietitian, take the time to select an RD with whom you feel comfortable and confident.

FOOD SOURCES OF IMPORTANT NUTRIENTS

NUTRIENT	FOOD SOURCES
VITAMIN A	Liver, fish-liver oil, fortified milk, eggs, carrots, dark-green leafy vegetables (e.g., spinach), yellow vegetables (e.g., sweet potatoes), yellow noncitrus fruits
VITAMIN B-1 (THIAMINE)	Whole-grain cereals, brewer's yeast, lean pork, legumes, seeds and nuts, enriched cereals
VITAMIN B-2 (RIBOFLAVIN)	Meats, poultry, fish, dairy products, enriched cereals, broccoli, asparagus, spinach
VITAMIN B-6 (PYRIDOXINE)	Chicken, fish, kidney, liver, pork, eggs, brown rice, soybeans, oats, whole-wheat products, peanuts, walnuts
VITAMIN B-12	Low-fat meats, fish, poultry
VITAMIN C	Green and red peppers, broccoli, spinach, tomatoes, potatoes, strawberries, citrus fruits
VITAMIN D	Fortified milk and margarine, eggs, butter
VITAMIN E	Vegetable oils, wheat germ, nuts, green leafy vegetables, whole-grain products

VITAMIN K	Green leafy vegetables, dairy products, eggs, fruits and vegetables, whole-grain cereals
FOLATE (FOLACIN)	Liver, yeast, dark-green leafy vegetables, legumes
NIACIN	Lean beef, poultry, fish, whole grains, enriched cereals
PANTOTHENIC ACID	Lean beef, poultry, fish, whole-grain cereals, legumes
CALCIUM	Dairy products, dark-green leafy vegetables (especially broccoli, kale, and collards), tofu, lime-processed tortillas, soft bones from sardines and salmon
IODINE	Seafood, dairy products, iodized salt
IRON	Lean meat, eggs, vegetables, enriched cereals, dried peas and beans
MAGNESIUM	Nuts, seeds, legumes, whole grains, dark-green leafy vegetables
PHOSPHORUS	Meats, dairy products, fish, poultry
POTASSIUM	All fruits and vegetables
SELENIUM	Seafoods, meats (especially kidney and liver), whole grains, seeds, nuts
ZINC	All animal products (especially lean meats, liver, eggs, shellfish)

RECOMMENDED DIETARY ALLOWANCES

FOOD AND NUTRITION BOARD, NATIONAL ACADEMY OF SCIENCES—NATIONAL RESEARCH COUNCIL

RECOMMENDED DIETARY ALLOWANCES,[a] Revised 1989

Designed for the maintenance of good nutrition of practically all healthy people in the United States

Category	Age (years) or Condition	Weight[b] (kg)	Weight[b] (lb)	Height[b] (cm)	Height[b] (in)	Protein (g)	Vitamin A (μg RE)[c]	Vitamin D (μg)[d]	Vitamin E (mg α-TE)[e]	Vitamin K (μg)
Infants	0.0–0.5	6	13	60	24	13	375	7.5	3	5
	0.5–1.0	9	20	71	28	14	375	10	4	10
Children	1–3	13	29	90	35	16	400	10	6	15
	4–6	20	44	112	44	24	500	10	7	20
	7–10	28	62	132	52	28	700	10	7	30
Males	11–14	45	99	157	62	45	1,000	10	10	45
	15–18	66	145	176	69	59	1,000	10	10	65
	19–24	72	160	177	70	58	1,000	10	10	70
	25–50	79	174	176	70	63	1,000	5	10	80
	51+	77	170	173	68	63	1,000	5	10	80
Females	11–14	46	101	157	62	46	800	10	8	45
	15–18	55	120	163	64	44	800	10	8	55
	19–24	58	128	164	65	46	800	10	8	60
	25–50	63	138	163	64	50	800	5	8	65
	51+	65	143	160	63	50	800	5	8	65
Pregnant						60	800	10	10	65
Lactating	1st 6 months					65	1,300	10	12	65
	2nd 6 months					62	1,200	10	11	65

[a] The allowances, expressed as average daily intakes over time, are intended to provide for individual variations among most normal persons as they live in the United States under usual environmental stresses. Diets should be based on a variety of common foods in order to provide other nutrients for which human requirements have been less well defined.

[b] Weights and heights of Reference Adults are actual medians for the U.S. population of the designated age, as reported by NHANES II. The median weights and heights of those under 19 years of age were taken from Hamill et al. (1979) (see pages 16–17). The use of these figures does not imply that the height-to-weight ratios are ideal.

[c] Retinol equivalents. 1 retinol equivalent = 1 μg retinol or 6 μg β-carotene.

[d] As cholecalciferol. 10 μg cholecalciferol = 400 IU of vitamin D.

[e] α-Tocopherol equivalents. 1 mg d-α tocopherol = 1 α-TE.

[f] 1 NE (niacin equivalent) is equal to 1 mg of niacin or 60 mg of dietary tryptophan.

273

		Water-Soluble Vitamins							
Category	Age (years) or Condition	Weight[b] (kg) (lb)	Height[b] (cm) (in)	Vitamin C (mg)	Thiamin (mg)	Riboflavin (mg)	Niacin (mg NE)[f]	Vitamin B₆ (mg)	Folate (μg)	Vitamin B₁₂ (μg)

Category	Age (years) or Condition	Weight[b] (kg)	(lb)	Height[b] (cm)	(in)	Vitamin C (mg)	Thiamin (mg)	Riboflavin (mg)	Niacin (mg NE)[f]	Vitamin B$_6$ (mg)	Folate (μg)	Vitamin B$_{12}$ (μg)
Infants	0.0–0.5	6	13	60	24	30	0.3	0.4	5	0.3	25	0.3
	0.5–1.0	9	20	71	28	35	0.4	0.5	6	0.6	35	0.5
Children	1–3	13	29	90	35	40	0.7	0.8	9	1.0	50	0.7
	4–6	20	44	112	44	45	0.9	1.1	12	1.1	75	1.0
	7–10	28	62	132	52	45	1.0	1.2	13	1.4	100	1.4
Males	11–14	45	99	157	62	50	1.3	1.5	17	1.7	150	2.0
	15–18	66	145	176	69	60	1.5	1.8	20	2.0	200	2.0
	19–24	72	160	177	70	60	1.5	1.7	19	2.0	200	2.0
	25–50	79	174	176	70	60	1.5	1.7	19	2.0	200	2.0
	51+	77	170	173	68	60	1.2	1.4	15	2.0	200	2.0
Females	11–14	46	101	157	62	50	1.1	1.3	15	1.4	150	2.0
	15–18	55	120	163	64	60	1.1	1.3	15	1.5	180	2.0
	19–24	58	128	164	65	60	1.1	1.3	15	1.6	180	2.0
	25–50	63	138	163	64	60	1.1	1.3	15	1.6	180	2.0
	51+	65	143	160	63	60	1.0	1.2	13	1.6	180	2.0
Pregnant						70	1.5	1.6	17	2.2	400	2.2
Lactating	1st 6 months					95	1.6	1.8	20	2.1	280	2.6
	2nd 6 months					90	1.6	1.7	20	2.1	260	2.6

Category	Age (years) or Condition	Weight[b] (kg)	(lb)	Height[b] (cm)	(in)	Calcium (mg)	Phosphorus (mg)	Magnesium (mg)	Iron (mg)	Zinc (mg)	Iodine (μg)	Selenium (μg)
						Minerals						
Infants	0.0–0.5	6	13	60	24	400	300	40	6	5	40	10
	0.5–1.0	9	20	71	28	600	500	60	10	5	50	15
Children	1–3	13	29	90	35	800	800	80	10	10	70	20
	4–6	20	44	112	44	800	800	120	10	10	90	20
	7–10	28	62	132	52	800	800	170	10	10	120	30
Males	11–14	45	99	157	62	1,200	1,200	270	12	15	150	40
	15–18	66	145	176	69	1,200	1,200	400	12	15	150	50
	19–24	72	160	177	70	1,200	1,200	350	10	15	150	70
	25–50	79	174	176	70	800	800	350	10	15	150	70
	51+	77	170	173	68	800	800	350	10	15	150	70
Females	11–14	46	101	157	62	1,200	1,200	280	15	12	150	45
	15–18	55	120	163	64	1,200	1,200	300	15	12	150	50
	19–24	58	128	164	65	1,200	1,200	280	15	12	150	55
	25–50	63	138	163	64	800	800	280	15	12	150	55
	51+	65	143	160	63	800	800	280	10	12	150	55
Pregnant						1,200	1,200	320	30	15	175	65
Lactating	1st 6 months					1,200	1,200	355	15	19	200	75
	2nd 6 months					1,200	1,200	340	15	16	200	75

METROPOLITAN LIFE INSURANCE COMPANY'S HEIGHT AND WEIGHT TABLES (1983)

MEN

Height (without shoes)		Small Frame Weight in Pounds (without shoes)	Medium Frame Weight in Pounds (without shoes)	Large Frame Weight in Pounds (without shoes)
Feet	Inches			
5	1	123–129	126–136	133–145
5	2	125–131	128–138	135–148
5	3	127–133	130–140	137–151
5	4	129–135	132–143	139–155
5	5	131–137	134–146	141–159
5	6	133–140	137–149	144–163
5	7	135–143	140–152	147–167
5	8	137–146	143–155	150–171
5	9	139–149	146–158	153–175
5	10	141–152	149–161	156–179
5	11	144–155	152–165	159–183
6	0	147–159	155–169	163–187
6	1	150–163	159–173	167–192
6	2	153–167	162–177	171–197
6	3	157–171	166–182	176–202

Statistical Bulletin, Metropolitan Life Insurance Company

WOMEN

Height (without shoes)		Small Frame Weight in Pounds (without shoes)	Medium Frame Weight in Pounds (without shoes)	Large Frame Weight in Pounds (without shoes)
Feet	Inches			
4	9	99–108	106–118	115–128
4	10	100–110	108–120	117–131
4	11	101–112	110–123	119–134
5	0	103–115	112–126	122–137
5	1	105–118	115–129	125–140
5	2	108–121	118–132	128–144
5	3	111–124	121–135	131–148
5	4	114–127	124–138	134–152
5	5	117–130	127–141	137–156
5	6	120–133	130–144	140–160
5	7	123–136	133–147	143–164
5	8	126–139	136–150	146–167
5	9	129–142	139–153	149–170
5	10	132–145	142–156	152–173

HOW TO DETERMINE YOUR BODY FRAME BY ELBOW BREADTH   To make a simple approximation of your frame size:

Extend your arm and bend the forearm upwards at a 90-degree angle. Keep the fingers straight and turn the inside of your wrist toward the body. Place the thumb and index finger of your other hand on the two prominent bones on either side of your elbow. Measure the space between your fingers against a ruler or a tape measure. (For the most accurate measurement, have your physician measure your elbow breadth with calipers.) Compare this measurement with the measurements shown below.

These tables list the elbow measurements for men and women of medium frame at various heights. Measurements lower than those listed indicate that you have a small frame while higher measurements indicate a large frame.

MEN

HEIGHT (In 1-inch heels)	ELBOW BREADTH (Inches)	HEIGHT (In 2.5-cm heels)	ELBOW BREADTH (Centimeters)
5'2"–5'3"	2½"–2⅞"	158–161	6.4–7.2
5'4"–5'7"	2⅝"–2⅞"	162–171	6.7–7.4
5'8"–5'11"	2¾"–3"	172–181	6.9–7.6
6'0"–6'3"	2¾"–3⅛"	182–191	7.1–7.8
6'4"	2⅞"–3¼"	192–193	7.4–8.1

WOMEN

HEIGHT (In 1-inch heels)	ELBOW BREADTH (Inches)	HEIGHT (In 2.5-cm heels)	ELBOW BREADTH (Centimeters)
4'10"–4'11"	2¼"–2½"	148–151	5.6–6.4
5'0"–5'3"	2¼"–2½"	152–161	5.8–6.5
5'4"–5'7"	2⅜"–2⅝"	162–171	5.9–6.6
5'8"–5'11"	2⅜"–2⅝"	172–181	6.1–6.8
6'0"	2½"–2¾"	182–183	6.2–6.9

Source of basic data: Data tape, HANES I—Anthropometry, goniometry, skeletal age, bone density, and cortical thickness, ages 1–74. National Health and Nutrition Examination Survey, 1971–75. National Center for Health Statistics.

Copyright 1983 Metropolitan Life Insurance Company.

Courtesy: Statistical Bulletin, Metropolitan Life Insurance Company.

REFERENCES TO SECOND OPINIONS

Should you wish to read the complete reviews and comments from which the Second Opinion sections in this book were excerpted, you may contact the appropriate sources listed here. Be sure to refer to the title, author, and publisher of the book(s) in which you are interested.

ALA BOOKLIST
The Professional Multimedia
Evaluation Service
American Library Association
50 East Huron Street
Chicago, Illinois 60611

AMERICAN HEALTH
MAGAZINE
80 Fifth Avenue
New York City, N.Y. 10011

CURRENT DIET REVIEW
P.O. Box 1914
Rialto, California 92377

ENVIRONMENTAL NUTRITION
NEWSLETTER
52 Riverside Drive
New York City, N.Y. 10024

HEALTH GAZETTE
P.O. Box 1786
Indianapolis, Indiana 46206

JOURNAL OF THE AMERICAN
DIETETIC ASSOCIATION
216 West Jackson Boulevard
(Suite 800)
Chicago, Illinois 60606-6995

JOURNAL OF NUTRITION
EDUCATION
428 East Preston Street
Baltimore, Maryland 21202

LIBRARY JOURNAL
245 West 17th Street
New York City, N.Y. 10011

LOWFAT LIFELINE NEWSLETTER
52 Condolea Court
Lake Oswego, Oregon 97034

NUTRITION AND THE M.D.
NEWSLETTER
14545 Friar (#106)
Van Nuys, California 91411

PUBLISHERS WEEKLY
249 West 17th Street
New York City, N.Y. 10011

ABOUT THE AUTHORS

Deralee Scanlon is a registered dietitian with expertise in a variety of die-tetic areas, including nutritional assessment, diet therapy, nutrition for senior citizens, and weight-loss counseling.

A nutrition authority for such broadcast media as Cable News Network (CNN), ABC-television and KABC TalkRadio, she has also written for several magazines and is the author of an earlier book, *The Wellness Book of I.B.S.*

Ms. Scanlon's weekly "Ask the Dietitian" newspaper column appears in a number of Southern California newspapers.

As a member of the National Speakers Association, Ms. Scanlon lectures to organizations and other groups on the subjects of nutrition for health, effective dieting, and consumer-awareness label reading. She also teaches a course on weight management and nutrition for seniors.

Larry Strauss is a writer who specializes in medical and science books. He is the co-author of *Growing Younger, When You Have Chest Pains, Financial Tips for Teachers,* and *What Do You Mean You Don't Want to Go to College?*